Praise for

I Dropped 142 lbs in a Year and Lost 220 lbs in a Day

Alicia I can not tell you how excited I am about you sharing your diet plan and seeing how well it worked for you. So far I have lost 11 lbs and looking forward to dropping at least 10 more following your plan. I have watched you walk those hills and push away sweets like it was a disease and I know I can do it too especially after seeing how much you shed those pounds...1, 2, 3 lbs at a time! Such an inspiration to me and my whole family.

Latondra Jackson

Alicia Ash has been a great inspiration for me. I met Alicia over a year ago and was very expressed by her motivation, determination, and consistency surrounding her weight loss. Her momentum and sense of urgency was very vital and played an important role in this phase of her life. After meeting Alicia, she encouraged me to want to lose weight "the normal way." There were times when I wanted to throw in the towel and give up but I would call Alicia and my strength was renewed. Thanks Alicia for being who you are...keep shining!

Much Love, Shanda 'Dee' Hixon

I would like to dedicate my thirty-four pound weight loss to Alicia Ashe. For the last ten years, I have struggled to obtain and maintain an optimal weight. It was not until I met Alicia that I met my personal goal and remained steadfast with my weight loss.

Alicia is an aspiring and motivating individual that truly touched my life in a special way. Alicia helped me develop and initiate a successful change in my lifestyle. Before I met Alicia, I was despondent and very miserable with my constant weight gain. I had tried several diets to lose weight but always failed after a couple of months. Alicia's lifestyle plan gave me a sense of hope and direction that I needed to be successful.

My lifestyle and diet change have truly altered my life. I no longer feel defeated and I have maintained a constant weight loss for two years. I have more energy than ever before. In addition to eating healthfully, I also exercise twice each week. According to Alicia, eating healthfully and exercising are both required to achieve and maintain desirable outcomes.

In closing, I would like to thank Alicia for her generous and giving spirit to share her success with me. Not only did she give me the special ingredients to lose weight, but she also gave a me a priceless, lifetime friendship.

Carmen Jackson Weeks

Alicia your weight loss has really inspired me, to lose my weight and find myself again. I have lost over 25lbs and going to continue through your success. Thanks for the encouragement.

Love Ya! Auntee Diane

Alisha Ash's story is a tremendous testimony of the power of self-motivation. Seeing her work tirelessly to drop the weight was phenomenal. When I met Alisha, she was at her peak in weight gain and to look at her now, it's so encouraging to me. The real highlight of her efforts came she appeared on national TV, The Oprah Show, demonstrating her accomplishments and natural beauty to the world. I would say this is a must read for anyone battling to beat the bulge.

Roslyn Giles

I have known Alicia for over 20 years and she has always been beautiful inside and out. I can remember back in our high school days we both had some insecurites about our weight. To see her go through this awesome transformation was such an inspiration to me. When I saw Alicia on the Oprah Show I immediately knew that whatever weight issues that I was facing, I too could overcome them. Alicia has inspired me to set goals for myself and I am on my way to a healthier me. I have one of her newspaper articles on my refrigerator as a reminder that I can control food, it does not have to control me.

Nichole Carthen-Jones

Having known Alicia Ash before and after her drastic weight loss I would have to say that her accomplishment has been a great example for myself and many other young adult women who struggle with being overweight. It has been a great encouragement that if you become discipline and believe in yourself, with Gods help all things are possible. Thanks for being the pattern.

Kristi Faison

Alicia has inspired me in more ways than one. She has motivated me to take the natural route of shedding this unwanted weight as well as encouraged me to face life with strength and courage. She is a true hero in my eyes and now the world will know also.

Petra Gertjegerdes
Arts & Entertainment Editor
Columbus Times Newspaper

How I Dropped 142 lbs In A Year & Lost 220 lbs In A Day

Alicia L. Ash

iUniverse, Inc.
New York   Bloomington

iUniverse books may be ordered through booksellers or by contacting:

iUniverse
1663 Liberty Drive
Bloomington, IN 47403
www.iuniverse.com
1-800-Authors (1-800-288-4677)

Because of the dynamic nature of the Internet, any Web addresses or links contained in this book may have changed since publication and may no longer be valid. The views expressed in this work are solely those of the author and do not necessarily reflect the views of the publisher, and the publisher hereby disclaims any responsibility for them.

ISBN: 978-1-4401-8188-7 (sc)
ISBN: 978-1-4401-8190-0 (ebook)
ISBN: 978-1-4401-8191-7 (hc)

Printed in the United States of America

iUniverse rev. date: 04/19/2010

Acknowledgements

I am grateful for each day God has given me and for Blessing me through this journey and with good health.

To my wonderful parents George and Zeytee Jones Thank you for never doubting me and constantly supporting me.

My grandparents Robert and Clester Turner, and the late Author & Sarah Joyner (I miss you so much)

To my beautiful children Ms Merceytee Jones and Laporche Hussey (my neice) You two have grown up to be amazing woman. Thank you for walking with me when I know there were days you did not want to (lol) and for believing in me and stepping up to the plate when I really needed you I love you. My son William Ash (trey) the apple of my eye, you are so amazing Thanks for keeping momie on track. I love you son. My sister Tonya Hussey, Elquan, Laquan and charles Hussey and also Jazzmen Wolfe Thank you Babies. To my best friends for putting up with me (smile) through this transformation.: It was not easy, but I do appreciate you Latondra Jackson my bff I love you girl) Tacala Hightower, Diane Neal (my auntie) Neytee Warren, Theresa Burden and Mr William Ash friends forever. Juanita Williams Rosalyn Giles and Gail Durden, and to my manager Mr Carlos Scott wow thank you so much for believing in me You are a Blessing from above.All the radio stations for putting the book on Blast Thank you Foxie 105 dj chip, Vicki James &mICHAEL Soul.and the one and only Michael Baisden. Ms Oprah Winfrey for having me on your show and you being my hero because of you I was able to believe in me again. Thankyou. Last but not least the Love of my life Mr Milton D Hamilton thankyou for being so amazingly supportive and understanding through this process and for reconizing and reflecting on my inner beauty which allowed me to let that flow outward. I deeply love appreciate you. Alicia Ash

Contents

FOREWARD
By: Angie Stone

As I wake up each day to another beautiful day that the Lord has blessed me to be on this earth, it doesn't take me long to realize that I am truly blessed to be here. I have two beautiful children who love their mother dearly, and I was blessed to have loving parents who likewise love me unconditionally. However, each second, minute, hour, and day that I am here, is a true testament to the will, power and most of all grace of God. You see, most people look at entertainers, celebrities or stars and only see the glitz and the glamour of fame and fortune. Rarely, if ever, do people have an opportunity to see entertainers as the average everyday people who we are. Sure, a lot of us get to travel around the world to places the average person can only read about or Google on the internet. Some of us even live in the biggest homes and drive the fanciest cars money can buy. Those are all great things to have and to be able to attain, but in the grand scheme of things they mean nothing in the eyes of the Lord, especially if you aren't using those resources for the betterment of his Kingdom and to do goodwill to you fellow brother or sister. I made a conscious decision several years ago that I would use my platform, fame and resources to bring national awareness to Diabetes and Diabetes testing.

Each year millions of people are affected by Diabetes and/or complications related to Diabetes. Thousands of those people eventually lose their lives to the disease each year. With that being said, Diabetes doesn't have to be the death sentence that we have made it to be. As a person who has been personally diagnosed with Type 2 Diabetes almost ten years ago, I am here as a living testimony and example that Diabetes doesn't have to be a death sentence. The first step in dealing with Diabetes is very simple. "GET TESTED" I can't stress enough the importance of getting tested to make certain you know what your glucose levels are. Getting tested gives you an opportunity to adjourn yourself accordingly, as far as your lifestyle is concerned. You may get tested and discover that you aren't Diabetic, but that you have higher than recommended glucose levels. With that information your doctor can now inform you on how to go about changing your diet to lower your glucose level. Unfortunately Diabetes drastically impacts the African-American community twice as hard as it does other races. One of the reasons why Diabetes is so prevalent in our community is directly related to our diet which has traditionally been high in fats and sugars that we eat on a routine basis. The reality is that most African-Americans are uninsured or underinsured and are also scared to go to the doctor. However, they aren't scared because of the health ramifications, but they are mostly afraid of being hit with an outrageous medical bill and the prospect of being stressed out by medical bill collectors trying to recoup their payment.

The second and thing you should do is "GET EDUCATED". I can't stress enough the importance of you, your family members and friends educating yourselves about the symptoms of Diabetes as well as various things you all can do to help prevent yourselves from getting

Diabetes. I hope that this book on Alicia Ash's life inspires you and motivates you to take claim over your life and get tested for Diabetes. Alicia story is a real life testimony of how you too can take claim and responsibility over your life and put your self in a position to lead a healthier and more quality lifestyle.

Prologue
Standing in the shadows.

Once again I was in the shadows. It's okay though. This would be the last time. I was in the darkness looking out through the curtains at the well lit stage. Holding court in the center of that loving light was Oprah. A woman that has reached such a pinnacle of power and success her one word name was more than enough to open any door. Clear any path. Publishing empires were built on her recommendation. Movies. The magazine. What part of mass communication did this woman not influence with the sheer magnetism of her influence?

Not one I could think of.

Breathe Alicia. Try to breathe. My heartbeat so strong I could feel it outside of my body. It was strange though. There was no uncomfortable sweat beading down my back. No feeling of faintness. Just this weird calmness as I stood in the shadows watching Oprah spin her magic with the effortless grace she had come to personify to me.

On stage the story of a weight loss journey was being spun. However, this time, the queen of hostesses got to add a new ingredient to the recipe of food battles. A happy ending. Oprah lost a lot of weight. She had a new lease on life and health as she showed off her new svelte body.

This was my moment. The moment that I've been waiting for. My chance.

I smoothed my hands down my front, skimming the silk of my blouse and linen in my skirt. What I felt was all sleek now. I went from fat to fine. My body was all feline grace now. The flatness of my stomach and curve of my waist reminding me of life in high school. My pride made me swell within the confines of these sexy clothes, my lungs gaining their first full intake of breath in what felt like hours.

Shadow dwelling I am about to bid you adieu.

Chapter One
I'm Fat and I Know It

It's been twenty-five years, and I still remember my first day of high school as if it was yesterday. September 1984. I was so excited that I could hardly sleep the night before. I remember waking up at 6 AM to get dressed. Just a short year ago, I didn't have a desire to get up at all. But on that day, however, my first day of high school, I woke up early with so much zest and zeal for life. Everything had to be perfect. Fresh starched jeans, beautiful red shirt with matching red pumps. My hair was long, black and curly. My size...a perfect size eight. I remember twirling around in the mirror. No, I wasn't vain. I just wanted to make sure that everything looked right. It was the first day of high school, and I knew it was the start of a new life for me. Little did I know then that I would never see that perfect size eight again until almost twenty-years later.

Weight had never been an issue for me. Maybe you could say that I had good genes. Or maybe it was just sheer luck. Who knows? My dad was in the military, and we were stationed in many different places. We moved around a lot. It seemed like as soon as I gained a new friend, one that I could trust, it was time to move again.

It was the story of my life. I became used to being the new girl. The girl that everybody judged. The girl that no one knew if she was black or biracial... I just made sure that I was the new, cool kid. It didn't matter how fair my skin was or how curly my hair was, to be "in", you had to be cool.

It was October, and my birthday was in a few weeks. I think I was more excited because my mom told me that on my birthday I could start wearing a little lip stick and very little eye shadow. All the girls were wearing makeup and I think I was the only one who wasn't. At least, that is what it felt like. I begged her for months and months and finally she agreed! Even if she hadn't agreed, I had my backup plan in place. I had a Caucasian friend whom I told that she should give me her eye shadow since her mom was cool, and she could get more. Not to mention, she would get the right kind.

So the next day she brought me all new makeup and said that her mom bought it for me. At that moment, I felt she had the best mom in the world. She was so lucky. Not that my mom wasn't great too but just not about makeup.

It was getting closer to my birthday, and I was counting down the days. I couldn't wait to wear my makeup. I was still in disbelief that my mom had agreed, so I was walking on eggshells around her. Praying she didn't take it back. I had done everything she had asked me to and then some.

I never understood why my sister was never into make up or high-heeled shoes. I wore pumps every day and she would only wear blue jeans and t-shirts. I would tell her all the time that she was not in the cool crowd. My sister Tonya was a grade ahead of me, but we were like night and day. We were so different. At the high school we attended, only the really cool people hung out down stairs and the nerds hung out upstairs. So when I arrived my freshman year, I was told that you don't hang out downstairs unless you are going to eat lunch. I had to hang out down there and everyone thought I was in the tenth grade. No need to change it. Finally, I was in the cool group. Makeup, high-heels. Go Alicia go! Not to mention at school, I was the center of attention with all the boys. They loved themselves some me. Heck, I was in love with me too.

At home, I started having the big head. I had forgotten that school was not home. At home, I was Alicia. Wash the dishes, take out the trash, clean your room Alicia. Not the miss cute Alicia who all the guys worshipped and the girls wanted to hang out with.

One day my mom said look here sweetie you are a beautiful girl but your nasty attitude makes you ugly and you best straighten it. At the time, I couldn't even begin to fathom why my attitude would make me ugly. What was my mom talking about? I was too cute to be ugly—ever!

When all my friends got a job and started buying their own clothes, I had to do the same thing. Yes, I wasn't real original back in those days. I told my mom that I wanted to work so that I could buy my own clothes. My mom agreed under one condition. I had to keep my grades up. Easy enough, I though.

After some searching, I finally got a job at Taco Bell. I worked every day because I learned that the more hours that I worked, the more money I made. The more money I made, the more clothes and makeup I could buy. The more clothes and makeup I bought, the better I looked and the more I stayed in with the cool kids. I was living the good life. In fact, I was so sharp that some of my teachers had started to ask to borrow my clothes, but my mom didn't play the clothes sharing. In fact, we weren't allowed to spend the night at anyone else's house either. This was true especially if she didn't know their parents. Heck, even if she knew their parents, it was still a tough sell.

Keeping my grades up, working and then I started modeling in different fashion shows. This was truly the highlight of my life. I thoroughly enjoyed modeling. This became my life. I loved all that modeling had to offer. It brought me a sense of self worth. Modeling validated my beauty. It meant to the world that you were certified pretty. I love d modeling clothes and having people clap. I could hear the whispers of how pretty I was. I was on top of the world.

I would either enter different contest or someone would enter me in a contest. Modeling felt like I was born to do it. Not only did I model but I could sing too. All anyone had to do was put a microphone in my hand I lit up like a Christmas tree.

I would go to the skating rink on the weekends and enter the singing contest and win every time. I won all the school talent shows too. I was on top of the world!

My world got even better when I met this guy named Bobby at the skating rink. He was there singing too. He sounded just like Prince. The boy could sing. I told Bobby about my connections at the radio stations and soon Bobby and I became a duo (music only). We started to sing and perform at various events. We opened shows for large events, dinners, clubs, etc. We even had a band that would play for us. I was living my dream. I had always wanted to be a performer. I loved every minute of it. How can I ever forget our signature song, "Secret Lovers" by Atlantic Star. When we performed that song, people were swaying in the audience. Some even accused us of lip singing because it sounded so authentic. Nope, no lip singing. We could sing, and we really loved it. I'm in a band and an opportunity to really do some big things in music and fashion. It was 1988 when my dad came home with the news that we were moving to Columbus, Georgia. I couldn't believe it. I had a boyfriend that I loved. We had been together for three years. I didn't want to pack up and move and start over. No way. I was devastated. I cried for days. I told my friends and they cried with me too. I knew that I would never ever marry anyone in the military because it was a life that I was already fed up with.

4

Chapter Two
I Did Not Want To Move

April 1988- Columbus, GA. We moved and got settled fairly quickly. We moved so much that moving was an art form for my family. In fact, in most cases, our house was completely setup within a week. If you came by you would think we had been living there for years. Pictures on the walls and accessories completely in place.

Shortly after we moved in, my boyfriend caught the bus here to see me. Of course, I thought this was very cool. So, I told my mom she should let me catch the bus to see him for Christmas. Of course, my mom thought this was not cool. In fact, it wasn't even up for discussion. Her answer was a flat "no". But a no wasn't going to stand in the way of me and the boy I loved.

So, when Christmas came I decided would just plan my own trip. Big mistake. I thought that I planned it pretty well—at the time. I called the bus station to see what time the bus left. Correction. I called to see what time the late bus left. I wanted to plan my escape while they were asleep.

During that time there was a young girl that had moved in—25 years old and with a car. She was cool though. I asked her if she would take me to the bus station at midnight. She agreed.

It was 4 AM when my parents got up and realized that I was not in that bed. They called my boyfriend first. And by the time he got to the bus station to pick me up, his first words were, "your mom is driving down here to whip your A--."

I quickly got on the phone with my mom and after much begging, pleading, and crying, I convinced my mom to let me ride the bus back. She even agreed to let me ride the bus every now and then to see my friends.

I eventually got me a job at Taco Bell in Columbus and things started to change because I was older and more mature and meeting new people and realizing I wanted to date. I had only dated on person all through high school and he was a whole bus ride away! We were seventeen and engaged. What was I thinking? So, I started to get scared and started to date other people.

He was in college and joined the military went to basic training and was on the way, and I was at Taco Bell, looking cute and thinking I am not going to be tied down. I liked the attention that I received from all the guys. I was still a perfect size 8, and I looked fabulous.

His plan for us was to go into the military, since this was a huge military town. He thought that he could make a lot of money in the military and our lives would be set. We would get married and live a good life.

Next thing I know, he dropped out of college, joined the military, and was on his way to see me! Me...the same me who was having a ball dating OTHER guys. I wanted to be sure that he was the one and what better way than to date to make sure. The problem is that I was on a date with my new boyfriend when he pulled into our driveway. We had just gone out to eat. I noticed the strange car in the driveway, but I thought it was just one of my dad's military friends. Yes, the tag was out of town, but the tag is always an out of town tag. So, I did not think anything of it.

In we walk, laughing and talking after coming back from dinner and straight into the face of my fiancé! He was sitting on the couch with one of his friends. I could not say anything, so all I could muster was an unintelligible "excuse me" and walk past him into my parent's room.

My dad did not hold back on me. He told me that I was wrong and that I needed to handle it. I walk back into the living room and my fiancé asks that he and I go outside to talk. As soon as we step outside, I start to apologize profusely. I am talking, crying and apologizing all at the same time. In the middle of my tirade, my Columbus boyfriend comes out to tell me that I need to make a choice.

I tried to work it out with my fiancé. We made a go of it, but after a while and with the distance, we did finally break up. I continued to see the Columbus boyfriend. As a result, we began to see each other every day.

I see him for a very long time. We spent a lot of time together. A lot of time. So much time that when I start to complain to my friends about having a headache and feeling tired, they automatically assumed that I was pregnant.

Chapter Three
Where It All Begins

I got the test, took it, and sure enough.... I was pregnant. Everyone was so excited. I was still a little in shock. I am happy but in shock. Mostly, I couldn't stand to look at the father anymore. I wanted to hurt him. I wanted revenge. I asked my friend to pray for me everyday because I needed prayer! I actually wanted to hurt this man. I could not believe my emotions could be on such a rollercoaster ride. How one minute, I could think about him and nothing else and the next I wanted to erase ever knowing him. I once told my friend that I wanted to cut him just to see if he would bleed. She was on the floor laughing. Her exact words were, "with your scared self, you won't even step on a bug let alone cut someone."

Of course, I would not cut anyone and probably would not step on a bug either... but I did tell him to get out and I will call him when the baby is born. The funny thing was that I was not even a full two months and I was already trying to get rid of him. Actually, it was not him. He had not done much—except get me pregnant. However, the old adage goes, it takes two to tango. So, he wasn't the only one to blame. I was a willing participant. It wasn't him. It was just his scent. I could not believe that all the stuff that I have heard women talk about in the beauty shop was true... morning sickness, emotions on a roller coaster and scents driving you wild. I had all of that and more!

I was literally sick every day. At that time, I swore that I would not have any more kids. I kept praying that if God blessed me with a healthy baby boy, I would never have any more kids. I was going to get my tubes tied.

I was in the bed all day long. It took a while but eventually, I started to feel better. But it took a while to get there.

I had been so sick that I had almost forgotten that Valentines Day was here. My sister called and asked if I would come over and cut her twin boys hair before their grandmother came to pick them up. I am a little slow, not knowing that she was having a party that night. When I walk in, there are five people already there. So I just go straight to the bedroom to get in there and out of her way.

By the time I was done and cleaned the boys up and came out, there were quite a few people out there. I was really in no mood to socialize. So I spoke and told my sister to call me tomorrow.

I was trying to leave when this one guy started coming towards me. I keep walking towards outside. So does him. When we get outside, I told him that I am not interested and to take a good look at my pregnant belly.

He kept walking me to the car and insisted on having my name. He kept talking to me about him and where he was from and why he was at the party in the first place. He had just come in from Korea and some friends invited him to the party. He said someone told him to come so they could hook him up with some chick, as he put it. So why was he out here bothering me, I thought.

He told me that he was supposed to be at the party to meet her but he would rather "meet" me. I reiterated my pregnant belly by pointing to it while stating the words, "I am pregnant and not interested." He asked if I was married or dating someone. I told him that I was single.

Well, I must have been just standing there looking thirsty because the next thing I know we are pulling up at the store and he goes in and gets a 2 liter for us. He said, "I want to make sure if you get thirsty later, you are taken care of." I drove him back to my sister's house, and expressed my appreciation for the 2 liter. I asked his name. He said that everyone called him by his last name. Ash. I said, "Thanks for the drink Ash." He asked for my number and I gave it to him but one condition—that I could have his too.

We started talking every day. He wanted to make sure me and the baby was Ok. Now the question was, what did I want? I was fresh out of a relationship but he sure was cute.

Chapter Four
My Friend

Ash and I became the very best of friends. I had never met someone so funny in my life. He could make a dead man laugh. He was so hilarious. We would go out to dinner almost every night. He took me for banana splits, dessert, something different every day. And boy was the weight piling on, but I didn't care. I was happy. Pregnant and happy!

I just believed that I could lose it because I was pregnant. He never even cared about how big I was getting. He would always tell me how beautiful I was. I was just so amazed because here is a handsome, young man who is spending all his time with a woman who is carrying the baby of another man! Ash just said that he loved me and my long, black, naturally curly hair and my round, peach shaped face. He loved me for me.

Ash was a part of my life, and I loved it. He was military and would have to go to the field for 30 days at a time. He always called to tell me where he was. Before he headed out to the field, he would call me and tell me to come and get his truck and his credit card. He insisted that I got the things that I needed for the baby. I was still in shock and how freehearted this man was!

All my friends wanted to know if he had a brother. They couldn't believe how Ash had come into my life and just changed it for the better. So, I got dressed and went out to his unit to get his truck. I was feeling like maybe I should not take his credit card but he insisted that he would take care of me and my baby. I was not going to argue with him. He knew what he wanted to do, and at this point, I needed the help.

Since I had gained so much weight, I was unable to wear shoes. I had to wear slippers. I couldn't go to anyone's job if I wanted to. I felt like a fat pig. I kept telling myself that after the baby, I will get the weight off. I had to keep telling myself something because I was starting to become depressed. I had never looked or felt this way ever in my life. Remember me? The model and the perfect size 8. Gone

Instead of focusing on my weight, I turned all my attention and energy towards the baby. I start to setup my baby's furniture but I can't really do what I want to because I am living at my mom's house. Instead of a pity party, I made lemonade. I used what I had and made it very pretty.

Two weeks went by, and I was very ready for the baby. I had done all the decorating that I could do. I had made it nice and pretty. I was still feeling depressed, but I had to shake it off. I had to remind myself that the baby is coming soon and all things will change. I will start to look like my old self, and I am bringing a new life into the world. I had a new man and all is right with the world. I said that to myself as often as I could. The only problem is that I said but wasn't sure if I believed it.

Ash had been gone for two weeks, and I felt like I was getting bigger and bigger. I was trying not to stress out about it. To help calm my nerves, I started to go to bed earlier and earlier. I would wake up pretty early in the mornings, and I would always go straight to my mom's bedroom. Same routine every morning but one morning I went in to say good morning, my whole world changed.

Chapter Five
My Life Has Changed

I said my normal good morning to my mom, and she immediately jumped out of bed and looked at me in disbelief. "What is wrong with your face," she said. I didn't know what she was talking about, so I went to her dresser and looked into the mirror. Oh my God! I couldn't believe what I saw... my mouth was twisted and my face just looked horrible! What in the world had happened?

My mom is rushing around me, putting on clothes and trying to help me get ready. I am still frozen and she looks at me and says, "Alicia, I think you've had a stroke, and I am taking you to the hospital." A stroke. A stroke? A stroke. I am trying to digest the words and also think at the same time. I am pregnant. Why in the world would I have a stroke?

I stare into the mirror and just couldn't believe the image that I saw back. It was me in my clothes but it definitely was not my face. The peach face that I had grown accustomed to looking at was gone. I had had a stroke and now I wasn't just fat, but my pretty face was gone too.

When we arrived at the hospital, they decided to keep me. I stayed in the hospital for two weeks. I was still in a whirlwind of disbelief when they discharged me.

I came home with the reality that I may have some facial damage. Okay now its time for the real saints to start praying. I called all the prayer warriors that I knew and solicited their prayers. I was just wondering if I could get any worse. What if my face didn't return to normal? Would my friends treat me any differently.... Oh my God! What was Ash going to say or do? Would he continue to date me?

One of Ash's friends found out that I was in the hospital, and he gets word to him. As soon as he gets in, he comes directly to my house. I was so ashamed about my looks that I couldn't even look at hi. I kept my hand over my mouth. I did not want him to see how messed up my face was. I was afraid that if he saw me, he would leave and never come back. I looked that badly.

True to who has always been, Ash put his arms around me and told me "It's okay baby, don't worry about your face. You are still beautiful to me." At this point, I am very emotional. I couldn't do anything but cry. I cried because I knew he just had to pity me. How could he love me like this? I cried because he must love me enough to lie to me. Truth is told, I was just crying because I needed to let it out.

The next day Ash called me and said get dressed because we were going to the mall. Instantly, I told him no. I wasn't going to the mall. I couldn't let the general public see me this way. There was no way. He simply said to get dressed and he would pick me up in two hours.

I got dressed but putting on my makeup was a challenge. I was trying to put it on without looking into the mirror. For the first time in my life, I had no desire to look into a mirror or apply makeup. I thought back to when I was a teenager and had begged my mom to wear lipstick and makeup. Funny how things come full circle.

I started to put on my lipstick. My right lip was so twisted that it could almost touch my nose. I used my long hair to my advantage. I pulled my hair over my right side to take away the attention from my face.

I have gotten so fat that I did not wear pants at all. I had put on a nice skirt, a really big shirt, and my white Isotoner slippers. I dressed for comfort. Fashion Alicia was gone.

We are in the mall and Ash is holding my hand as if he was not aware of the people staring at me. Or maybe it was in my head. I felt like everyone was looking at me. He never let go of my hand. He kept my hand in his and held on to it tightly. We even stopped and had lunch.

I started feeling really tired. So, after lunch, I told Ash that I needed to go and lay down. The next day was my baby shower, so I needed to get plenty of rest.

On the day of the shower, my mom was hostess and so many people came with so many gifts. I could not believe it. My daughter's godmother Marion bought so many clothes. It was amazing. I did not have to buy the baby a thing. It was a blessing. I had so much fun at the shower, but I did start to get really tired. It must have shown in my face and my actions because everyone told me to go and lay down. Most of them teased that the baby was probably due very soon. Little did I know at the time, they were right. Within the next few days, I was in labor.

Chapter Six
Married And With A Baby

"Pop!" This was the sound I heard before my water broke. I immediately told my mom. Thank God for her! I told her that I was going to take a shower. My mom laughed and said, "Girl, you can not take a shower. You are going to the hospital."

We arrived at the hospital, and I was in labor for almost 30 hours. 30 hours that was a miserable feeling. Finally, they decided to do a c-section. Finally, my baby girl comes out. She had a cone head from being in the birth canal so long with no water. Oh God, what is wrong with my baby's head? The nurse reassured me. She told me to calm down. She assured me that my baby's head would not stay that way. I was so thankful for my new baby girl. The world was perfect.

Two months later Ash got sick, and I mean really sick. For a few days we thought he had the flu. He took all the flu medicine that we could find. Nothing helped. It happened to be my birthday weekend and I had planned to go out with a few friends. However, my mom pulled me to the side and told me that I had better take Ash to the emergency room since he was still not looking so good.

No sooner than we arrived at the hospital, Ash passed out. It really scared me. What scared me worse was when his blood started to come through is skin. I was panicking. I had never seen anything like this before. What in the world could be wrong with him?

Apparently, it was a new one for the doctors too because they flew in a specialist from Washington, DC. The specialist examined him and gave me the worst news of my life—Ash was not going to make it. He was in the final stage of spinal meningitis.

I called his parents. Of course, they immediately started planning to make the trip. I called anyone and everyone who I thought knew the true power of prayer. We needed a miracle straight from above. I respected what the doctors had to say but I knew that it was not over until God said that it was. I expected and believed God for a miracle.

They put Ash in ICU, and no one could go in but me and his parents. In a matter of a few weeks, he started to change for the better. Even though, he had to stay in the hospital for another month, we knew God had healed him. Most cases of meningitis end in death. Praise God for our blessing!

Even though I had just had a new baby, I was still at the hospital every day. I think after a week of him getting out of the hospital he asked me to marry him and I had just had a baby but still was at the hospital every single day. In just that short instance, we had become a true family. We were there for each other in the good and the bad times. I was so thankful that Ash was healthy and my baby girl as well. God had blessed me beyond words.

Our wedding was nothing elaborate. We went to the courthouse and immediately settled into our first apartment. I didn't care about a big wedding. I was married to my best friend. The man that I would spend the rest of my life with. He had been my knight in shining armor. Finally, things were settling down again and my life was starting to slow down enough where I could enjoy it. I was married. It had taken a bit to get there, but I was married.

One day while enjoying married life, I got a call about my paternal grandmother. She had been sick off and on. This time it was different. I was told that I needed to come down immediately. She lived about an hour and a half drive away. I called my husband at work, and he prepared to take me down.

Before we could leave, I got the call that she had passed away. I just fell on my knees. I could not believe it. I hadn't slacked up on my eating habits and this sent me over the edge. I was eating every bit of bad news that I had ever received. Ash being sick, the stroke, the weight gain, my grandmother's death. I was constantly eating and didn't even notice that I was doing that.

I was determined to be strong for my dad. He was the spitting image of my grandmother. I had noticed it before but now he really looked like her. I guess it was a combination of being around him and all our relatives that made me notice it even more.

We arrived at the funeral, and my uncle who had not seen me since I put on all the weight, walked over to me in shock. I could see the look of surprise all over his face. He gave me a hug and shook my husband's hand. He called me by my nickname of penny but makes the joke that he is going to have to change that to fifty cents. Even though I smiled, the joke really hurt. It hurt me so much. Thankfully, Ash didn't find it funny either and his look said so.

That night, I went home and took a good look at myself in the mirror. I was so depressed. What had happened to me? I used to be a perfect size 8. I was a model. I had curves. I had fashion. I had style. I was not this woman who didn't even wear pants anymore. I used to wear a pear of jeans and even the women had to look twice. What happened to the perfect size 8 Alicia?

Chapter Seven
Low Self-Esteem — What You Do

Most women lose some of the weight gained during pregnancy, but I didn't lose any. At the time, I was 4'11, weighing 237 pounds. I figured that I was not a pretty sight. I didn't like to look at myself in the mirror. How in the world could Ash want to look at me? I had started to rationalize that if Ash wanted a divorce, I wouldn't be upset with him. After all, I had been telling him that I would lose the weight. I told him that it was all baby fat. Now, I had no excuse. The fat just was not coming off.

Ash never complained, though. When his company had picnics, I told him to go without me. I did not feel good because I did not want to go out in a skirt looking crazy. I was a size 22. I was a long ways from that perfect size 8.

As a big girl, I felt I had to do more to be hot, like keep my hair done, makeup and nails looking good all the time. I took extra care on my face. My goal was to make my face as cute as I could, so hopefully the rest of me would not matter as much. You know how people are always saying, "she has a cute face." At that point, I longed for that compliment. I had to have people say something positive about me. I needed it.

As things would go, when you are on a roll, you are on a roll. My husband received orders to relocate to Fort Riley, Kansas. I knew I should not have of married a military man. Of course, I did not want to go. I had moved most of my life and was tired of moving. I wanted to stay close to my mom and my family. Ash was not having it.

My husband tells me that we were going as a family, and we are not separating. He tells me that my parents can visit and the move will not be such a bad thing. I started to feel a little better about it, but my mom began to develop health problems. I was afraid to leave her when she needed me most. In fact, the thought of us leaving sent her to the hospital. Her blood pressure was so high; she had to stay in the hospital for a week.

I still had to leave. We put off our moving a couple of days, just until she was released from the hospital. I think I ate during the entire trip to Kansas. I was so worried and depressed about my mother. I am convinced I can't take too much at one time it. I was severely depressed, to the point where I was sick. Food was becoming my refuge for anything and everything. I was eating constantly. When I thought about my mom, I ate. When I thought about not being near her, I ate. When I thought about how far it was between her and me, I ate. I ate all the time. I was getting bigger and bigger. I was out of control.

We arrived at Fort Riley and stayed at a hotel for two weeks, just long enough to get a place of our own and get settled in. I immediately figured out my new plan. Being far away from home was not as bad as I thought it would be. I figured I would lose the weight while I was away, then surprise everyone when I visited.

We lived in a townhouse, so my plan was to start by running the steps in my home everyday, because I refused to take my fat butt outside in a skirt. So, the first few days, I figure if I eat just once a day, I will automatically lose weight because I'm not eating as much. My plan backfired – by noon, I was starving. I was starving beyond belief.

I ran those stairs for two days. On the third day, I went up the stairs two times. When I went back up the stairs for the third time, I could see my bed from the corner of my eye. When I got to the last step, I went straight to bed and told my daughter go downstairs and bring the cookies. It was time for All My Children. So much for my plan.

As hard as I tried, I just could not do it. I hated that I couldn't be normal and wear a sweat suit to workout outside like everyone else. I just felt so insecure in a sweat suit. Not to mention, I could not find one that was flattering in any way. I felt like the blimp in anything. I refused to go outside. I needed to be indoors to work out. My plan was to work out as hard as I could and then surprise everyone. I was just too insecure to go outside and really work off the pounds.

I will admit that a couple of times, I thought I would be better off dead, but every time I had those thoughts, I saw the face of by beautiful daughter. I had to live for her. The sad thing was that she was the only reason that I had a desire to live for. I was so depressed. I just could not take much more of my life.

Photo Gallery

Before

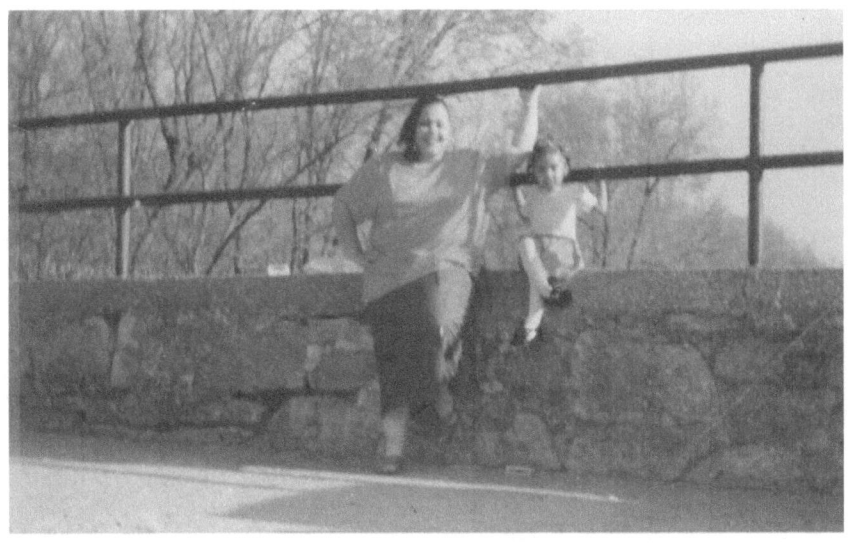

Me and my daughter, Ft. Riley, Kansas going to see the Buffalos, boy and I feel like one.

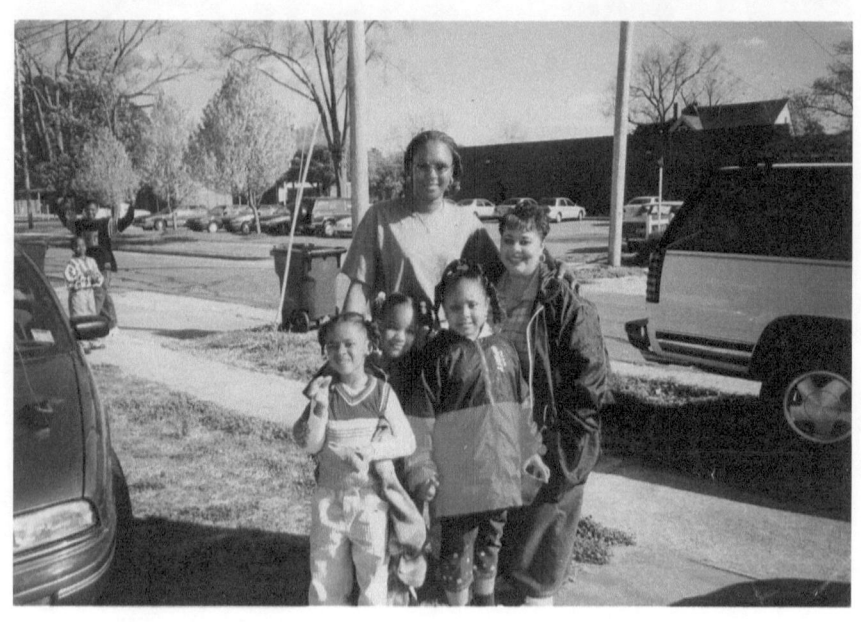

Visiting friends in North Carolina. I am really trying to hide behind everyone.

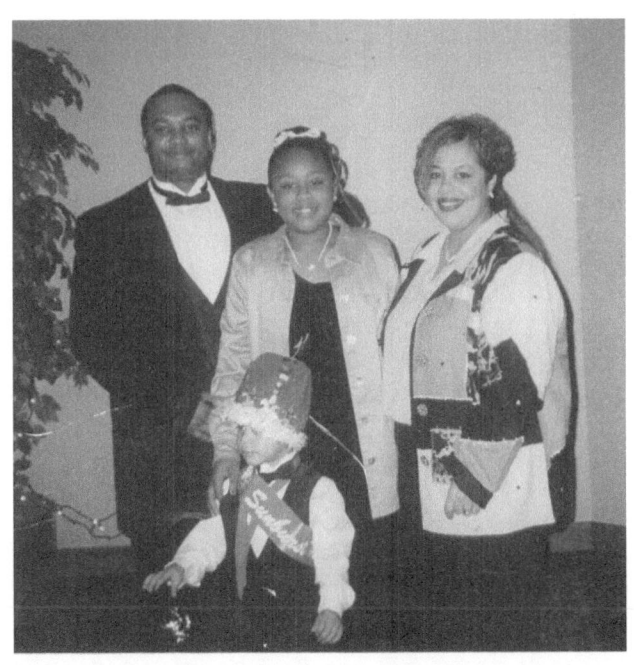

Me and the kids and ex-husband.
My son was crowned king in modeling competition.
Happy for him, but I was so miserable.

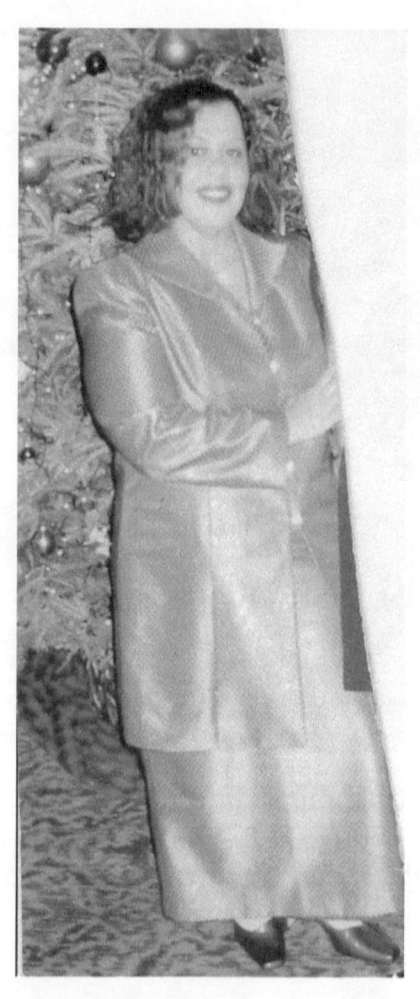

After

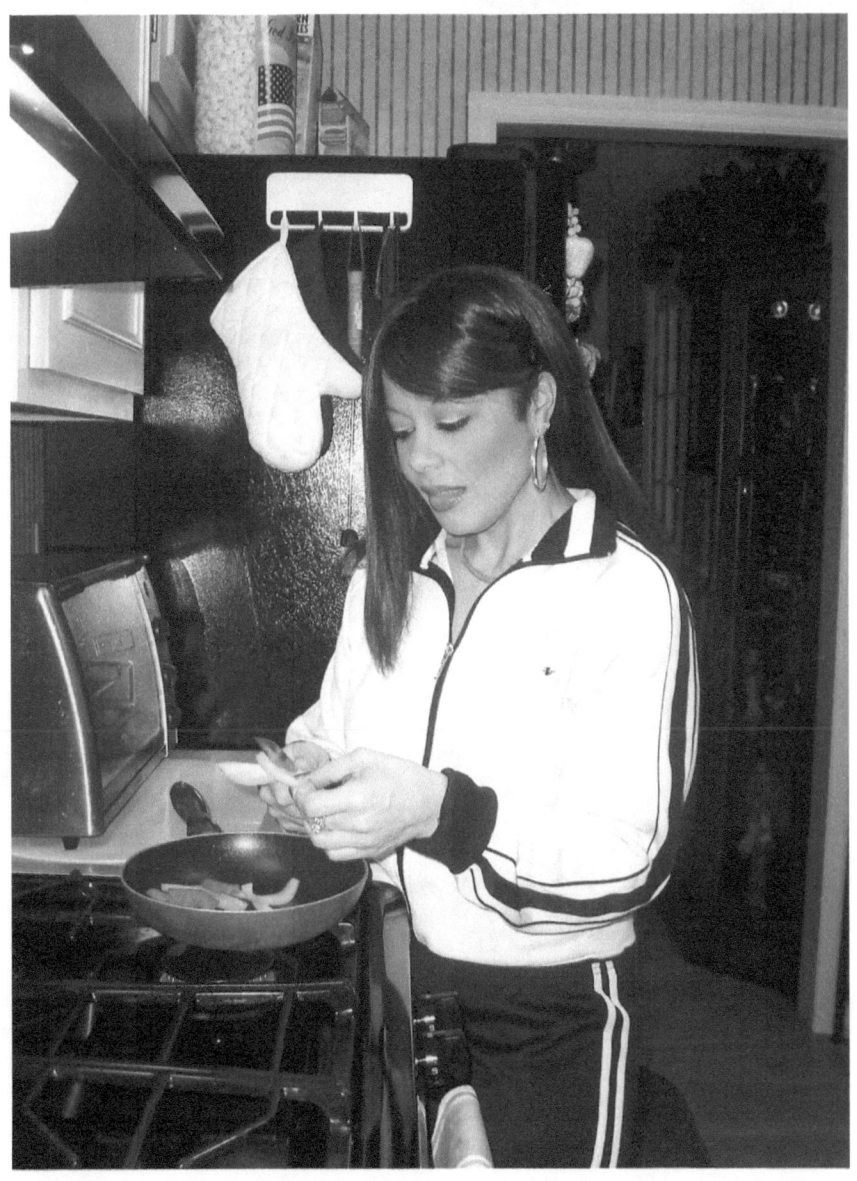

Eating healthy is a life-style I won't ever change.

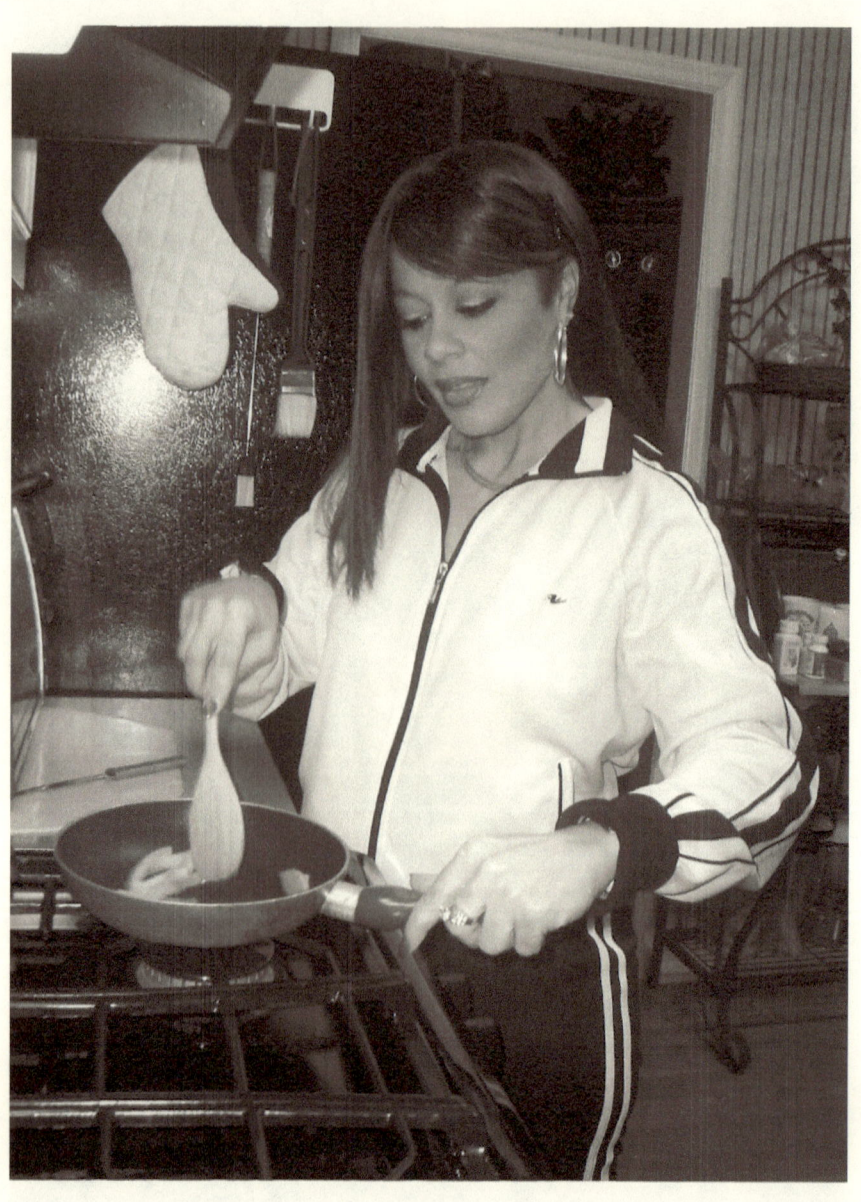

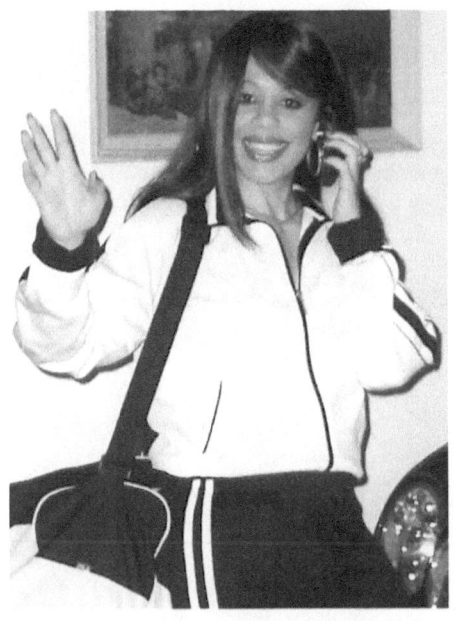

Excited that I am on my way to the gym. I never thought I would ever be excited about the gym.

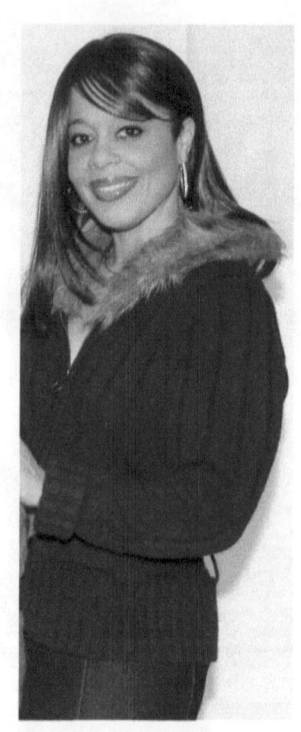

Although I am at my goal weight of 130. It was never about a size. It was about feeling good on the inside so that would flow outward.

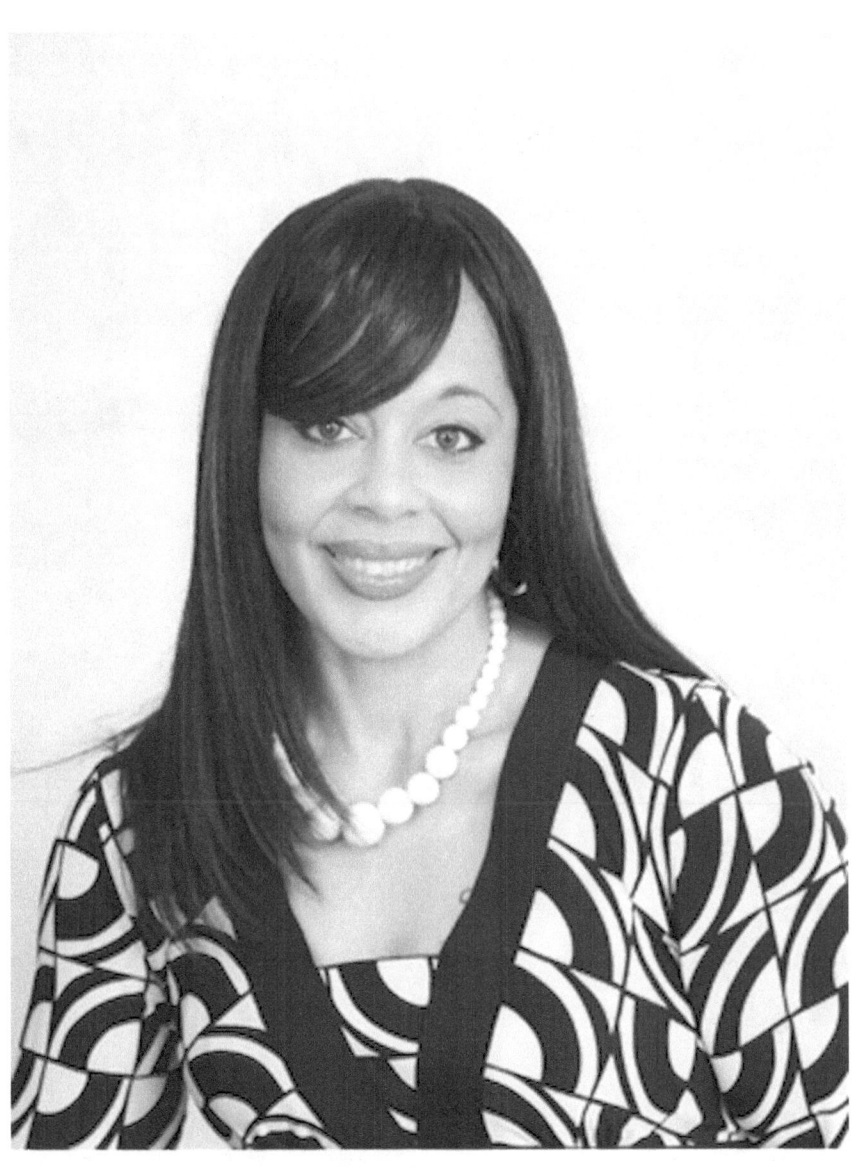

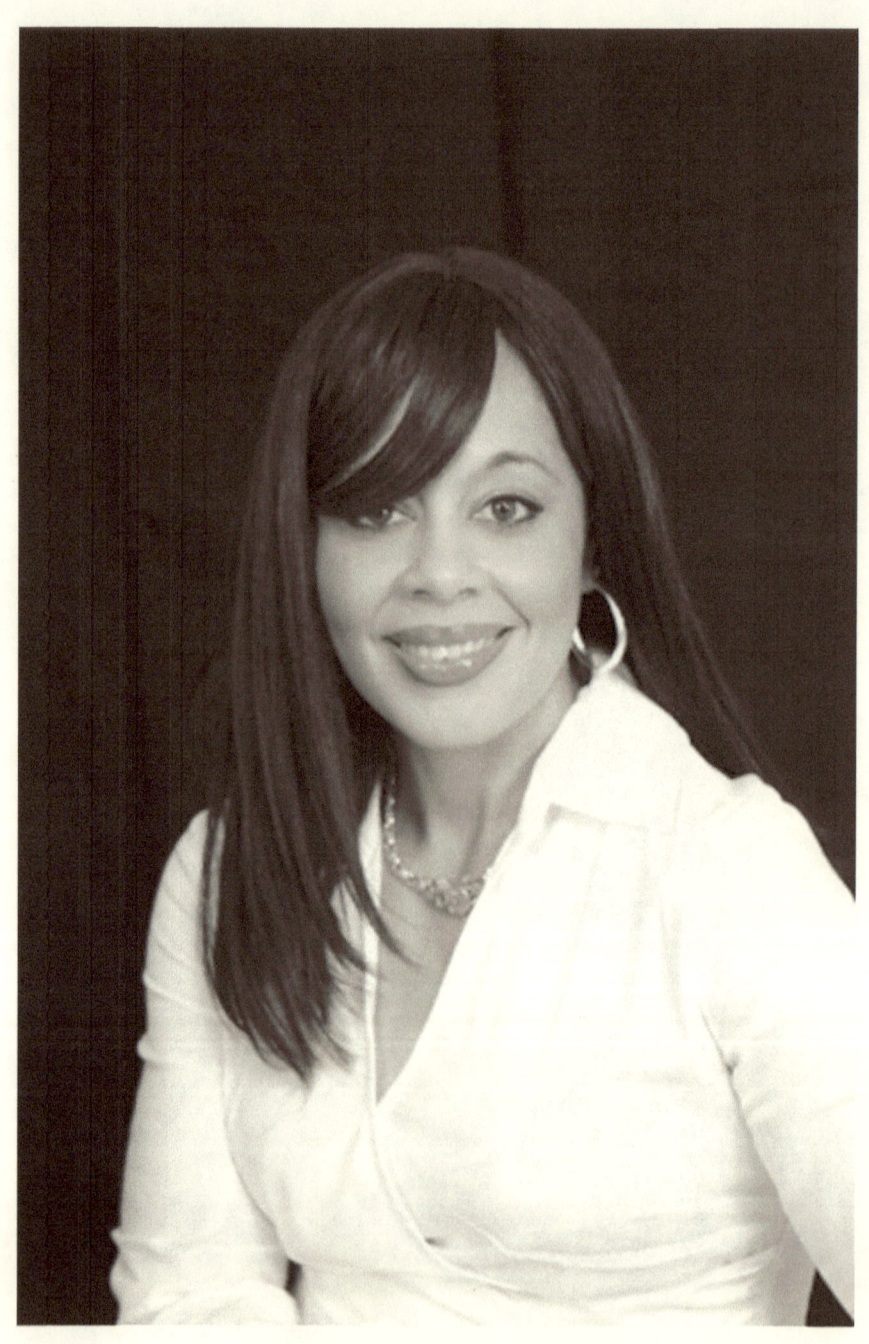

The me I knew I could be.

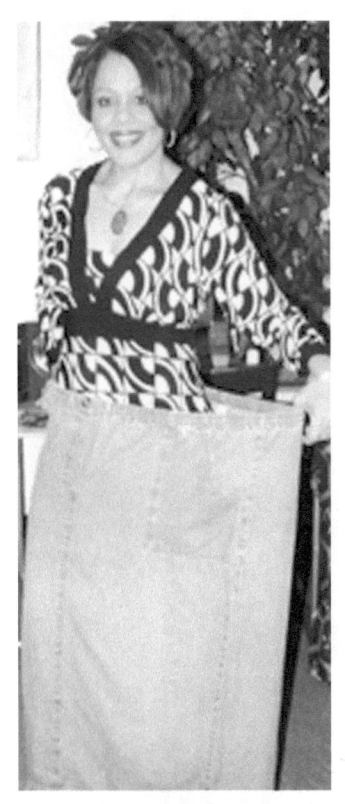

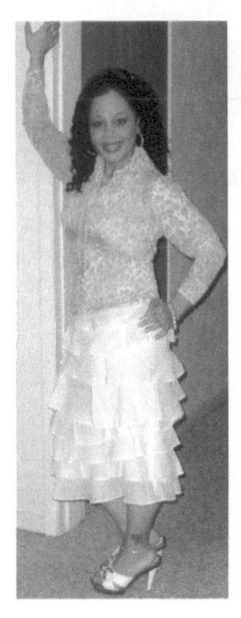

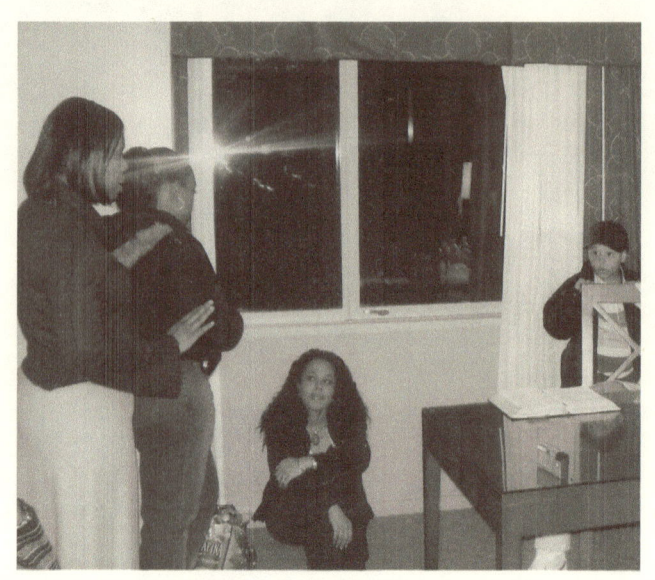

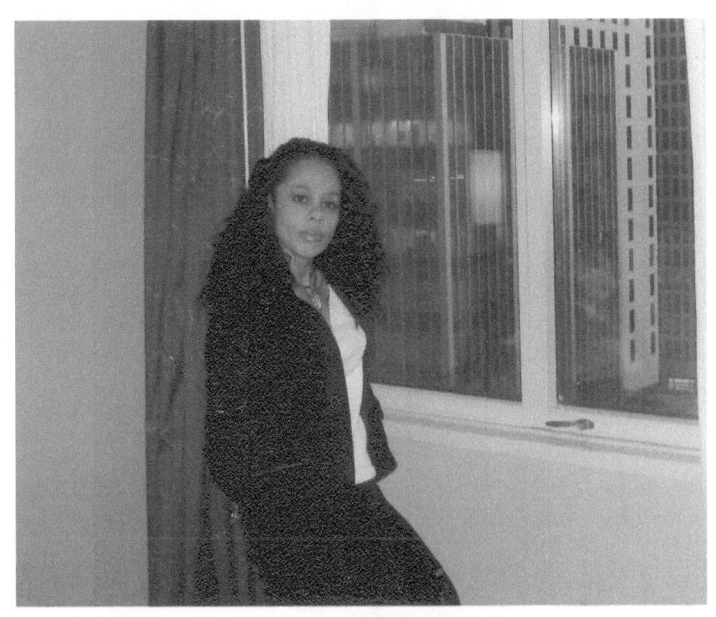

It is a journey but well worth it.

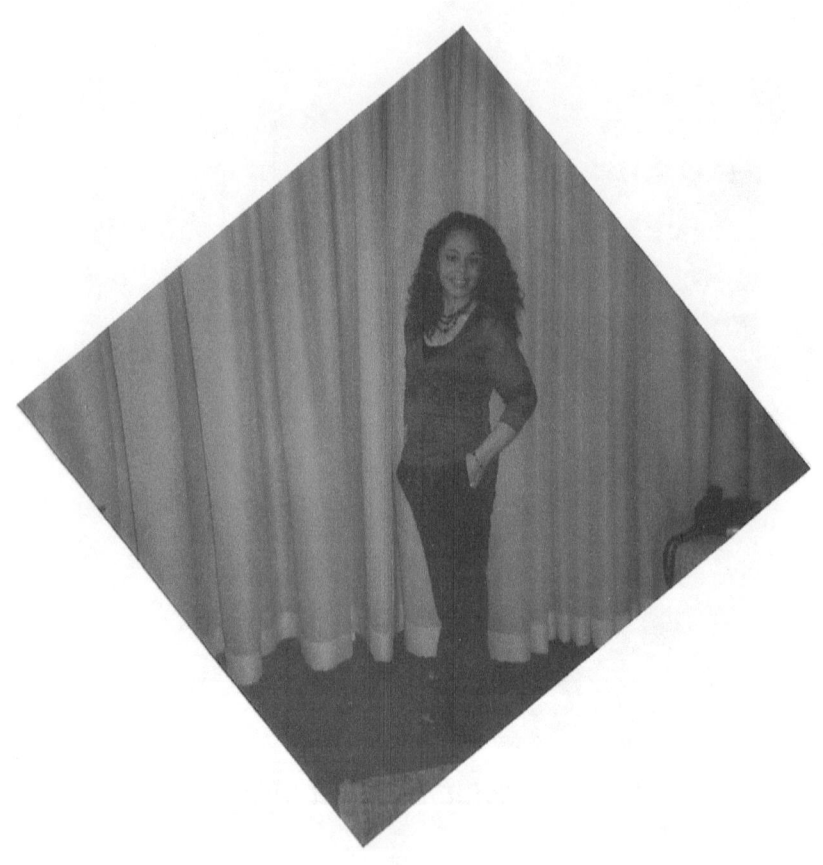

*Happy knowing I can do anything I put my mind,
heart, and soul in it.*

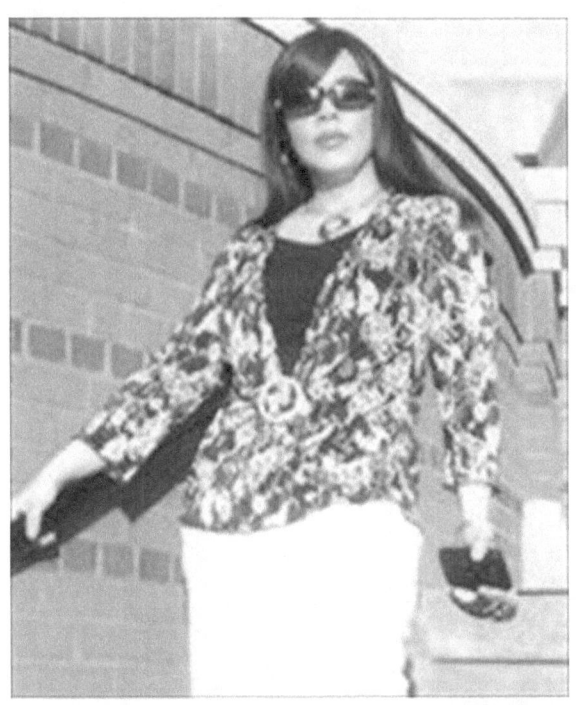

Taking my life back in a healthy way; mentally and physically not just for me but for my children.

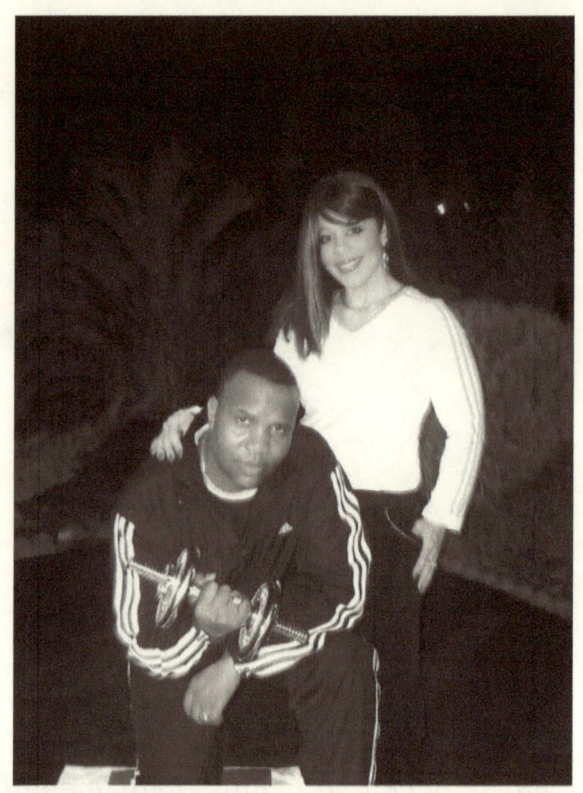

*Working out with my fiancé is always
a great motivation.*

Live, Love Life…This is My Mission in Life: To Give Back

My goals are to continue empowering, uplifting, and motivating others to their life goals, whether it be mental or physical well-being. My passion for personal development emerged during my own struggles with depression, surviving three mild strokes, obesity, low self-esteem, bankruptcy, being homeless and divorced. I overcame all those life-altering setbacks, and I knew I did not go through all that and not commit suicide without a purpose. I want to be able to come out and speak in front of so many with a smile turning my "why me" into a "why not?" Passion for others.

I will continue my commitment to myself and to improving the health of Americans by letting my voice be heard in schools, at social events, and in churches as well as through my book. My message is obesity is a silent killer and is linked to so many health problems that we are unaware of. I want to continue to get sponsors to help me push my foundation, SKIN DEEP, to not only help those who have lost weight and now have unwanted loose skin, but in turn help burn victims who need it. I also want to work on my clothing line, trAcedes, which is in the baby phase right now, but coming soon. Last, but not least, I want to be an inspirational and role model to unleash the greatness inside of you that I know is just waiting to come out. We all have it inside us, sometimes we just need someone to help pull it out.

Sometimes we don't even know that we are obese. We hide under the title of chubby or thick. We owe it to ourselves to own up to our true body type and realize that we would be much healthier minus the weight. When we begin to take ownership and responsibility for the bad decisions and eating choices, all learned or innate, we can change those habits for the better. Some facts on obesity are included in Appendix II..

I want to take some time and pull out the greatness in you. I wanted to share some of the letters that I've received over this journey and have included them in this book. I don't believe in keeping a blessing to myself. If I've been blessed, I like to pass it on. Believe it or not, these letters are cathartic for me. I want to share my experiences and gained knowledge with anyone who is willing to listen. I aspire to help others who are faced with the same issues I've gone through. I hope you enjoy the letters as much as I did answering them. They mean so much more to me than people even know.

Chapter Eight
I Don't Like Him

Ash was meeting new people at Fort Riley. He had a very outgoing and friendly personality. Before long, they were inviting us to participate in outgoing things. I never wanted to go because I already knew that I would be the biggest and the worst dressed person there. I felt like I was letting Ash down but I just could not go.

I remember one particular instance where we were invited to two retirement parties. Ash went into his closet, put on the first thing he puts his hand on, and looked sharp. I tried on ten outfits, just to get one that looked terrible. I was getting angrier and angrier as he walked by me looking so good. I was working extra hard on my hair and makeup to look halfway good. I'm thinking if he walks by the door one more time, I'm going to go off. I wanted to yell, "I can see that you look good, and I do not deserve you!" I was very depressed all the time. Why could not he see that and help me? But he was always so nice. I just wanted to cut the fat off my body and sew my skin back together.

My fat and depression were taking over my life. It was affecting my life with Ash. It was also affecting my life with my daughter. I knew she was unhappy because

I never took her to the park. I was too worried about someone staring at me. I would write out the grocery list and had my husband pick up the groceries. One of the neighbors went so far to ask if I were a vampire. He said, "Man she only comes out at night."

I felt like I was embarrassing him. We wanted to have a baby but couldn't figure out why I hadn't gotten pregnant. I was not on birth control, so I told him the problem must be on his end. I told him he needed to see a doctor, but he insisted that I needed to go.

I made an appointment, only for her to tell me that I was fat. She told me that if I lost the weight, I should have no problem conceiving. All I could think was, "I know this woman did not sit there and call me fat." My weight was affecting everything. I just knew my husband would leave me for sure now.

I walked through the office with tears in my eyes, embarrassed to tell my husband about the visit. As I opened the door, he was standing there already asking about the doctor's visit. That is when the tears really started to roll down my face. "Baby, what is it?" he said.

"She told me that I need to lose some weight."

"Ah, hell baby, let's go get a Whopper. It will be Okay baby."

I could not do anything but laugh at his silly self.

"If we have another baby, great. If not, that's Okay too."

I was really praying that I was pregnant. I would then have an excuse for being so fat. The fat was taking over my life. I needed to gain some control.

All the time in Kansas, I was supposed to be losing weight. Instead, all I had done nothing but eat too much. And then it was time for us to move back to Columbus, Georgia. I had to do something. I couldn't go back the same way I left. I felt like I had already let everyone down.

Ash, my daughter, my mom, and most of all myself. I had failed.

Chapter Nine
If One More Person Says
I Have a Pretty Face

I wanted a new look, so I began searching for the best beautician in Kansas.

"Look girl, I want a total new look," I told the stylist.

"OK, just let me hook you up."

The woman dyed my hair to a pretty brown and gave me an asymmetrical cut. I was so beautiful. I had a whole new look. Everywhere I went, people told me, "Oh my gosh, you have a beautiful face! Your hair is gorgeous!" Whew. I was back in business. I felt like I could distract people with my face again. I loved the fact that my face was enough that maybe no one would focus on the fat. But I had started to regret that too.

So, we prepared to return home to Columbus,GA. As soon as we got back to Columbus, I heard the same thing - "your face is so pretty."

I would rather they not say anything; because I felt like what they really meant to say was "your face is pretty, but you're fat as hell."

I really took offense to that, but my husband reminded me, "Baby, it's a compliment."

I just didn't like it. I didn't care what he was saying. I knew it was a backhanded compliment. I always hated how people felt like I should be thankful they said it. Or maybe I just felt like that. Who knows? My weight was affecting my mind.

We were finally getting settled in our new place. Thank God that this is the last time. We did not have to move anymore because my husband was now a disabled veteran. We could make Columbus our home.

Chapter Ten
I Need a Change

This is crazy. I have to take diet pills or something because yet again, I am the biggest one in our circle of friends. All of my friends were skinny or normal size. I had become the biggest one. I hated that. I felt like I was the one sticking out. Everyone else was wearing cute clothes, and I was still dressing like a blimp.

I had gone shopping and this woman asked me when was I due. I knew that I was big but not that big! I was mad and embarrassed all at the same time.

I had been searching for a job and didn't have much luck. Ash returned and found a job immediately. I felt like people just were not hiring me because I was fat. I could tell when I went on interviews. They were saying that I wasn't qualified or no openings but I knew it had to do with my weight. I just knew.

I saw an ad in the paper - no experience at all for the radio station. I was sure that I could do that. I got all cute, or so I thought I was anyways and went to the station. I go over there and the owner comes out and tells me to come on to the back so he can talk to me. So, I was thinking, "Okay, I bet he has not done this for anyone else." We sit down and he started asking me questions. Then all of a sudden, out of the blue, the guy said "I know I am a big guy, but my goodness - you are a really big girl."

I was stunned. I could not believe those words rolled of his tongue. I was so hurt and so embarrassed, but I was not going to tell anyone. That was the most hurtful thing any one could have told me that didn't know me.

I got my keys and my purse together while he was saying, "we cannot use you here." I told him thank you for lowering my self-esteem as I walked out the door. Needless to say, I slammed the door.

I got into my car and started crying. While I was driving to McDonald's to get a Big Mac meal, I ordered a large fry and an apple pie. I had to make myself feel better, somehow. It's like people think the bigger you are, the less of a heart you have. Damn, why are people so cruel?

I drove to the mall, parked and sat in my own pity, just wishing yet again that I was dead. I threw away the evidence and rolled down the windows so the car would not smell like food – Ash had told me that he was cooking. The fast food was just comfort food. The home cooked food was not going to get it. I needed to do some damage. I knew I didn't need the fast food, but I just didn't care. Everyone else was hurting me.

I got home and my husband told me to call my mom. It was very important. I was usually scared to call, so I just went over there. I got there and she was crying. I put my arms around her.

"Momma, what is it?"

She had to go on the kidney machine. I could not take that. My grandmother was on dialysis for a year, and it was not good. In addition to her having to take dialysis she was a diabetic and her blood pressure was extremely high. It seemed like it all happened over night. One day she was just fine, and then all of a sudden she was really sick.

I was not used to seeing my mom like that because she had always been the life of the party. She was always traveling. Always on the go. She went from being very mobile to immobile. This was not my mom. This really took a toll on me. Even her skin started to change. Her complexion had darkened because of the diabetes. Everything started changing on her. I put on another ten pounds. I really couldn't fit into anything now. I was the size of a hippo.

I had to find a job. But who was going to hire me as big as I was? That was going to be hard. I checked the paper, called and put in applications. No one called me. I waited and waited. I was a hard worker. So, what was the problem?

I started to feel really tired and I had a bad headache. I did not want to say anything about it but I needed to. So, I called my husband and my cousin who was an RN. She immediately thought that I was pregnant. "Girl, I am going to buy a test for you. I'm on my way."

She got there a few minutes after my husband. "Girl, I bought two, just to be sure." So, I went into the bathroom and did both test. I came out looking really sad, then I started smiling. "I'm pregnant!" We all started screaming because they knew how badly I wanted a baby. First, I said that we had to pray, and we did. We prayed and thanked God for our miracle.

The prospect of a baby changed my husband and my relationship. I started to act better towards him. I also thought he was treating me differently because he knew that I was miserable. Before the news of the baby, he had started to do things without me because he knew I would say no. I had been very angry with him, but we were starting to get close again.

On the day that we were going to find out the sex of the baby, I was ecstatic. It was the big day. As usual, I was late getting to the appointment. Ash was mad all the way there.

We got there and they tell us they would see me, but it would be in about 45 minutes. So, we wait and finally, they call me back there.

I am mad because he is mad. I looked at him as if to say, "Are you coming?" We both put on a happy face and proceeded into the doctor's office.

"Hello, Ash Family. What do you want this baby to be?" Like most mothers, I said healthy. Ash said he wanted a son.

The doctor moved the moved the wet sticky thing around on my stomach. Boy was it cold. The things women go through. If only men had to share in some of this. They would look at giving birth a little differently.

"Well, Mr. Ash, congratulations, man! You are having a son!" the doctor said.

That changed Ash's whole attitude. He actually had tears in his eyes. We were both very excited.

Funny how a little boy had changed how things were going between us.. I had been miserable. I had been resenting him like it was his fault that I was fat. My weight had really done a lot of damage to our marriage.

I didn't want to have sex. If I even thought he was going to roll over and touch me, I would just tell him my head hurt. I had to make up something. I just couldn't have him touching all of the fat. I knew he couldn't possibly be satisfied.

This would have us upset for a few days. I would try to apologize, but I just did not always feel like doing that. I was sorry, but I also expected him to understand my feelings. Big mistake. Men do not understand feelings. Men wanted sex. Especially a man who was used to having sex. I remember when we first met and how exciting our love life used to be.

I was not happy with my body, but I knew that I needed to concentrate on having a healthy baby. I was happy that I was having a baby, but I was wearing size

26 clothes. I was so big, I looked like someone blew me up, and I was about to pop.

It was so dangerous to be that big at only 4'11. My doctor was worried about my weight. I just didn't know what to do.

Since I had a C-section with my daughter, he let me pick my date to have my son. I chose July 2. At the baby shower, I was set for six months on clothes, diapers and everything. Everyone was so excited about this little boy. We decided to name him after my husband's father. He is William Ash III and his godmother gave him the nickname Trey.

There had to be about 30 people in the hospital waiting room. It was very exciting on Trey's birth day! When he came out, I cried because he looked just like me - same color, same curly black hair. He was so light; my friend passed him coming in to see me and asked "Where is the baby?"

I said you just passed him. "Girl that was a white baby. That was not him."

Trey was so adorable. People would go crazy over him. No matter where we went, he had an audience. The boy was a people person. My daughter, on the other hand, was laid-back and quiet.

Chapter Eleven
This Is When It All Begins

I had begun to realize that I wasn't going to find a job in the public eye and would not be able to wear a uniform. I was at an all time high of 267 pounds, and it was very unflattering. I was disgusting to myself.

I found some ads in the paper for house cleaning. That's me. I starched up my jean skirt, found a really nice shirt and went to the job interview. I pulled up in front of the house, and I was thinking to myself, "Oh, this house is not that big, I can do this."

I went in the house. It's like the house was dropped in the back, but it was so beautiful. It was a beautiful, modern home. The furnishings were all tastefully done. I could tell that the owner had great taste and a flair for decorating. The outside of the house definitely didn't match the inside of the home.

I told the lady if it's any consolation, if she was willing to come to my house right then to see how I lived, that is how I would take care of her home. She told me to fill the applications out.

"This is the first time someone invited me to see their house. The job is yours," she said.

I was so happy that I could still work and not be seen.

I would watch how this woman ate, cooked and what groceries she bought. They had a good lifestyle.

I paid close attention. I remember seeing soda in their house but apparently it was for guest only because no one drank it. Their sons did not even touch it.

The mother could be out shopping on the other side of the city but still she would come home just to fix a healthy meal for her family. They would have things like turkey sandwiches and apple slices. What a healthy way to eat!

Me, I would have pulled into the nearest hamburger place just as fast I could turn my wheel out of sheer convenience. I really admired the woman and her family. The way she fed her family was truly a new approach to me. I had never been around anyone who did not eat fast food. This became a big deal to me. It was then I knew that I had to change how I ate and lived. I wanted a new lifestyle.

At that time, I still had not taken full responsibility. I was still making up excuses. I made an appointment with my doctor and I told him I believed I'm so fat because maybe I had thyroids.

He said, "Mrs. Ash, we ran all those test for you the last time you were here. There is nothing wrong with your thyroids."

Then I start explaining to him, "Okay, something is wrong because my hair is starting to thin and my finger tips are always freezing cold. I have these mood swings like crazy and my skin is dry."

He said "Okay, that could be something else."

He made me an appointment to go see a specialist. I learned that I was border-line diabetic. I had to go on the same medicine my parents were on for diabetes.

"You should lose a little weight on these. Most people that take this actually lose weight, but I still want you to see the nutritionist," he said.

I started taking the medicine, and I did not lose one pound. Not one at all. I didn't even lose a ½ pound. I couldn't believe it. I had been excited to see some improvement. When there was none, I was very disappointed. No, I was mad!

I decided to ask my doctor if I could have the surgery. I was taken aback when he told me no. His answer for me was to go and hit the track, eat less, and watch what I ate! Who did he think he was?

Was this some kind of joke? I knew people who were getting the surgery. Why couldn't I get the same surgery? I needed some help! It felt like no one was listening to me. No one!

I had become a prisoner in my own home. It was home where I truly felt free. No more wearing a tight girdle. I could walk around free. I just let it all hang out at home. I was sick of wearing the contraptions that only made me look like I had lost 2 pounds. Not to mention, I could

The thing that got me was the few people I knew who had lost weight. I would try to get answers from them as to how they did. Funny how people want to keep a secret when they had succeeded at something. But when they were in search of answers just like me, they were doing the same thing I was—begging for answers from anyone and everyone.

"Oh, I just changed how I eat," they would lie.

"Girl, you mean to tell me that is all you done --you have lost over five or six dress sizes," I would say, hoping to get some information.

I wanted to know everything and people would not tell me. I hated going to trainers who had never been fat. They couldn't relate to the pain and anguish.

I was really convinced that I needed to stick with my 'out-of-sight, out-of-mind' thing I had going on in my life. I was also noticing that I was very testy. Everyone and everything was getting on my nerves. I hated running into people. In the grocery store, I cringed any time that I ran into someone that I knew. I would put a fake smile and say a quick hi, praying they didn't want to engage in conversation.

"Hey, Girl. I haven't seen you in a long time," I would say.

Sometimes we would chat for a few minutes and most conversations would result in them inviting me to their church. I would lie and say that me and Ash would visit, but of course, I had no intention of visiting ever. I didn't look forward to going to new places. I especially didn't want to go to someone else's church. It would just be a new group of people staring at me. At least that is how I felt.

I came home and somehow I did mention this church to Ash, and he said that we should go. His rationale was that it was only 2 minutes away from our house.

The woman was acting like this church was so amazing so come get a word. We went in the church. At the time, the name was Faith Worship Center. I heard the praise team singing. I thought it was the choir, but they had a praise team AND a choir. I could not believe the voices I was hearing. I was truly blessed through the song. After a few songs and a few other announcements, I was like "Okay, is the pastor coming out anytime soon?"

She got on that stage. She was beautiful. My husband and I looked at each other and were like "Oh, Lord."

The woman opened her mouth that day, and I understood what people meant by getting "got" at church.

We continued to go often, and I left that place full every time the doors were opened. I wanted to be there because I was so hungry for the Word. I knew something was missing - I just did not know what.

I was so moved, I called my grandmother and told her about the church. I asked her to come with me. I knew she was going to say no because she lives almost two hours away.

She said "Okay, if it is the Lord's will, I'll be there."

I thought she was so excited that her granddaughter was in the church house, she had to witness this for herself. Now my grandmother was from the old school. She had certain views and beliefs about the church. She didn't really believe in women pastors but she definitely didn't think one should be in pants. I just hoped and prayed that she enjoyed the word more than she cared about my pastor's attire.

We got in there and my grandmother and family were so moved by the praise team. I knew that pastor was getting ready to take the mic. Sure enough, she had on a black pantsuit. I was watching my grandmother out of the corner of my eye. At first, she hadn't said one word. In fact, she had barely moved but the next thing I knew, she was standing up saying Amen. Whoa! I did not know what she was thinking. After church, we all went to dinner, and she said, "Wow, the Lord used that woman preaching the word."

We joined the church and that really changed and amazed me because I felt like I was finally getting some control over my life. I had been searching to fill a void. I needed to fill an emptiness. I knew the Lord would fill. I now had a spiritual connection. Things were starting to line up. I felt like I could take on anything. I had God on my side. God had started to take my puzzle pieces and make them fit in ways I never knew they could.

One day for no reason, I was really feeling tired. I had this really bad headache. This was not the first time that I felt like this. I knew what was going on with my body. I limped slowly into the kitchen to get me some water and the cup fell out of my hand.

I called for my daughter. "Please call Theresa. I am really sick."

Chapter Twelve
Third Stroke

"I need help."

"She is on her way, momma. Do you want me to call dad?"

"Yes, let him know."

Theresa was on her way to take me to the hospital.

Ash worked like a hour and twenty minutes away. He got there in thirty minutes.

By the time I got to the hospital, Theresa had me so scared. She is a true drama queen.

"Oh my God! Your lip is twisted all the way up," she cries. So, they checked a few things and immediately put me in ICU and I started crying like oh God, You do have my attention now.

All of a sudden, this nurse walked in. She was so pure, she was like an angel. She leaned over to me and asked, "How are you feeling?" I still had tears in my eyes.

"Sweetheart, if you do not lose weight, your next stoke might not be a light one," she said with a voice filled with concern and love.

She walked out the room. I had no clue where she was going. She came to the window with Trey in her arms and Ceytee beside her. They were not allowed in the room, but Ceytee had tears rolling down her beautiful face. Trey was waving to me, not having a clue where we were. Felt like I was waving goodbye. She came back in.

"If you do not lose that weight baby, you are not going to be here to raise those beautiful children."

I never saw her again. I knew in my heart that she was right.

"Lord, if you let me make it out of this hospital, please give me the wisdom and the knowledge and understanding on where to even begin to lose this weight in a healthy way. I do not want to look sixteen again - I just want to be healthy."

I did not tell anyone but my husband. When I got out the hospital, I took it easy for a while, but I had started planning in my mind what I was going to do. I bought every magazine I saw that had a weight loss story on the cover. I wanted to know what was working, where they were successful in keeping the weight off. I literally became a weight loss researcher. This became my life for almost a year before I even began to put any of the information I learned into action.

Chapter Thirteen
My Story

I knew that I was going to do it because I knew this time, if I was going to make this work, I had to remember one thing - I had to retrain myself on how to eat.

I knew that any bad lifestyle you are accustomed to is a hard habit to break. I loved to write. So, I wrote down every one of my favorite foods - my weakness - and what a typical day is for me. I then began researching what would be the healthiest foods to replace those with.

I made a photo album with different methods I thought would come in handy to help me. Then I started going to the library. I checked out 14-16 books out at a time, extending my times to keeping the books and taking notes.

I started checking out workout tapes because I knew with any pregnancy you must exercise.

As much as I hated to exercise, I didn't have any pants to wear. I had made up my mind to lose the weight. I did not say I was confident, but this is a process.

I took this on as a crawl-before-you-walk method. I had a back-up plan for setbacks, for anything that would hinder me from being successful in taking back my life. I went to the store, and I bought a pair of sweat pants, sneakers, strength cords, and weight bar and hid it all in my closet.

I was so excited knowing my life was getting ready to change. I was still journaling and taking before pictures. It was like the Lord was giving me step-by-step guidance on what to do. Yet, I still had not started but was eager to do so.

We received in the mail a form that had my son's name on it for this little modeling competition. I was a little scared about it because I myself had been in so many, but my husband and I decided why not put him in there. Before I did though, I asked MerCeytee if she wanted to do it. She was a basketball player all the way.

So we put Trey in it. He won. He had different levels, and he kept winning them.

Eventually it starts getting bigger and bigger. Some of the competitions were in Atlanta. Trey's smile would light up a whole room. Eventually, we received a better offer from an agency inviting him up for a meeting. We went to the meeting. Little did we know, there were about 50 other children at the meeting. We all went in and the man talks about the company and told us what they were looking for ---basically he wanted the child not to be clingy and can follow directions well. His request was to speak to each and every child in the room individually. He wanted to see what they were made of. He asked who wanted to go first, and Trey's little hand shot up. I looked at Ash, and we were surprised that out of all the children, Trey was the only one willing to go in front of all those people. But I looked over and Trey has his hands so high up he was the only one that was willing to go in front of all those people.

Trey gets up and the man says, "You a nice looking fellow. What is your name?"

"William Lee Ash III, but they call me Trey."

"Why do they call you Trey?"

"I really do not know. They have been calling me that since I came out my mom's stomach."

Every adult laughed. He told Trey to do a few things, like dance. He did it all with a smile. I was amazed. He told him you are perfect for this business. He had to come back and do other things with the agency before he got a contract. Eventually he did get the contract. I was so proud of him.

If you are not in shape and cute, it was hard. There was a lot of traveling back and forth, but it was great experience.

In the midst of the traveling back and forth to Atlanta, my husband decided to buy a new house. That was music to my ears because I was ready to decorate a new house. He had already done all the work; we just had to find a house. We spoke with an agent and she asked me what I liked. My husband looked at me. "We want to be able to eat out, so you might want to ask me what kind of house we are looking for."

We went to see about ten homes. None of them came close. I knew what I wanted to live in. I also knew that those were not it. The realtor said that there was more to choose from if I like. There was one in particular that she thought I would like. Of course, it cost more but she knew I would love it.

She picked us up both the next evening. We were both eager to go.. I got off work early to cook and be ready. She picked us up. We arrived at the house. All I could is that whoever had it, had some really big dogs. The backyard was torn up. Ash kept saying that we could fix that.

The house itself was really beautiful - it was perfect. Ash told her that we wanted it. The realtor started to write up a contract. I was trying to get a deal. I told her that we would get it if they replaced the wallpaper, installed new carpet, and paid all the closing costs.

"Mrs. Ash, they are not going to do that. Do you want to risk your chance of another contract getting the house?"

"Can you please submit it?"

Me and Ash got in the car.

"Alicia, if you do not get that house, I am going to be mad," was the first thing out of Ash's mouth.

"We are getting the house. Do not worry."

He called all morning. "Did she call yet?"

"No. no and no. I will call you," I warned.

I will admit that I that I had started to get a little nervous.

She called me at 4:59 p.m.

"Mrs. Ash, I do not know who you know, but they agreed to everything you asked."

"Thank you, Jesus!" We closed on the house on my birthday. I was so excited!

Ash got out there in that yard every day. We lived on a corner lot, over a half acre. The grass was so pretty, it really looked like carpet.

We got Yard of the Month at least three times that year. He worked so hard. I did not think he was going to do it. I was all too shocked.

We were all settled in. I must admit, I took my time and decorated this house on a different scale of how I would normally do it.

If I could say so myself, I did my thing! People would bring other people by just to see our house. One lady told me that I should do it for a living. I was flattered.

"You are too funny, girl. This is just a hobby," I said.

"You should do this for a living," she insisted.

"Maybe in the future."

I would move furniture around during the eight hours that my husband was at work.

He would ask, "Who helped you?"

"I moved the refrigerator on the opposite side of the kitchen because it's a cut out for the fridge to go in."

I wanted to make an office in the kitchen, so I put a desk in there, hung a mirror over it and put a lamp shelf, it looked like a small office. It was cute and different. Most of the time, people have the right items, but have them in the wrong place.

I called one of my friends I had not talked to in a while. This girl is so funny; we always have a great time together. The great thing about us is we can go a couple of months without talking because we both knew how busy we are. I told her to come over.

"Girl, we just bought a house not too far from you."

She comes in with a fitted style tank top and some shorts on. She had lost so much weight. I was screaming. I couldn't believe how great she looked. I was very happy for her.

"Girl, how did you do it?"

She told me that we didn't live far from each other and we could walk together everyday. You are right up the street from me. We can walk together everyday. At first, I am thrilled, but I forgot I am still 267 pounds and I don't wear pants.

I just told her "Girl, you know I'm not wearing no pants."

"Come on girl; be at my house at eight in the morning. Alicia, do not be late."

So I went over there. This girl was walking so fast and kept yelling "Come on girl, you can do it!"

I said "Look, either you taking giant steps 'because you are 5'10, or I am really out of shape. Hell to the no - I will walk by myself."

"Come on girl," she prodded.

"Oh no, I am serious. Plus, I am really embarrassed. Everybody riding by on their way to work. I can't do it. Thanks girl," I conceded.

I went home and Ceytee and I decided we were going to the mall. We left Trey at home to work in the yard with his daddy.

I kept feeling like something bad was going to happen. I just did not feel right. But we stayed in the mall about three hours. On our way back home, we were cruising along in our red Expedition. We had just bought it.

All of a sudden, traffic slows. I looked through my review mirror and all saw was this big tow truck still going really fast and not trying to stop. I cannot move because there is traffic coming up on the other side. All I can do was put my arms over my daughter to make sure that she didn't go out of the truck. He hit me so hard, knocked my truck ten feet up into another car. He told the police that he reached down to pick up some paper and did not see the traffic had stopped. The ambulance had to come and get me. I was shaking uncontrollably. My back was hurting so bad.

I had to go to therapy for about three months. That messed up my plan on my weight loss.

Wow it's almost Valentines Day and our church was having a married couples Valentine's Dinner, and we were asked to speak. I was not happy with how I looked.

"I am not speaking, baby. You do it," I told Ash.

"They asked us to speak, baby. Look, just give a small introduction on us. How many kids we have and how long we been married. Just something simple like that, and I will take it from there," he said.

Leading up to the event, Ash had been praying and fasting for what to say. He walked in that night with this small bag in his hand. I asked what is in the bag. He insisted that he had bought the Dawsons - who asked us to speak - a small gift.

They introduced us. I was nervous, looking like a swollen hippo. I felt like everyone was staring. I kept thinking, why didn't I say no. I did my little part. And it was little. My girlfriend said, "I sneezed and you were done. Did you even say good evening, Saints?"

Next it was my husband's turn. I will tell you, he had the entire church in tears - men to even the pastor -

talking about the journey of our marriage, how he almost died, I stood by him and he is the man of our house. He spoke about my vision that I had for our lives.

Deacon Dawson handed him the bag.

"Baby, if you can accept these baby carrots for your eyes to continue to have the vision, then I pray you will accept this two karat ring for your finger."

I couldn't do anything but cry with every one else.

"You had to be praying for that one, because that was deep." I told him. Wow, I didn't see that one coming.

Shortly, after that event, were planning a surprise party for Ash. My mom was helping me plan the party. She got on my nerves so badly. I was like "Momma, are you going through menopause? You really need to ask your doctor for the patch."

Being brought up in the church and around my grandmother, Mrs. Clester Turner and her neighbor Gladys Mathis, I knew what real Christians were. My grandmother and Ms. Mathis were real Christians.

I used to think that they had God's phone number - they knew everything.

When I say they have been best friends forever, I mean forever. I had never seen them get upset with each other, never let a curse word slip out of their mouth. Nothing. I was a Christian, but every now and then, especially if you mess with a woman, especially a Black woman's kids, you will be told off. It's like we cannot handle that.

One time, my high school teacher saw my mom in Wal-Mart. At first, it was a hey how are you? Alicia is such a sweet girl. Blah. Blah. Blah. Then, she started telling her that I sat in class looking in the mirror all day. She also told her that I had an attitude. And of course, it was on then. My mom showed no mercy on her. Zeytee Jones will tell you off and you will not even know it until she's walked off.

I said that I will do better after living with my mom. I was able to see myself and I didn't want my husband or my daughter to see me as a bitch. Because I know that is not me, because I was so miserable and unhappy with myself, I had begun to take it out on other people.

During this time, I had bought a grand piano. I had a friend to come play the entire party. I had people come sing. Trey sang. Ceytee and Porsche said a poem. I had a friend to write a poem. I wrote her what we had been through and what she meant to me. That girl wrote a poem that had everyone in the room crying. I could hardly read the poem. I had it laminated and put in a very nice frame. My pastor had Trey get her some tissue. She said, "I do not know how much more I can take of this."

Those were happy tears, but when you are able to show someone how much you appreciate them, it is always great. Like my mom always said. "Give me my flowers while I'm living."

That night, my niece talks to me about living with me. She was about to be a senior and needed the help. I talked to Ash, and we agreed she was like our daughter. In fact, everybody at our church always thought I had three kids. She was truly like my daughter. So, she did live with us. That girl knew that she had me wrapped around her fingers. She kept moping around, saying everyone had a car and she really wanted one. I went out to find her a car. Ash begged me to not get a $2,300 dollar car. Do not get into debt. I did not listen. I bought her a car and she was so happy.

Chapter Fourteen
The New Me

I had to do something. I came from a family of high blood pressure, diabetes, strokes, heart attack, high cholesterol and kidney failure. So many generational curses.

I knew in my mind that I needed to stop it at me and not pass that down any more generations. If you are from the south, you know it's famous for good southern food like collard greens, ham hocks, black-eye peas, neck bones, potato salad, candied yams, fried chicken, cornbread, banana pudding, sweet tea and Kool Aid. One thing for sure in our house, if nothing else, we always ate very well.

My dad, Mr. George Jones, he did not play that. On payday, we would get up early Saturday morning. He would cook eggs, cheese grits, bacon, sausage, biscuits and orange juice. When he knocked on your door one time, you best get up and go wash your face, brush your teeth and be at the table. If you looked like you did not do both, he would make you go back and do it. We all had to eat at the table together, then get ready to go the grocery store. My sister Tonya never wanted to go, but that's fine by me because I am the baby and daddy's girl. That meant I could sit in the front and get what I wanted.

It never failed. He would spend about 200 dollars or more on groceries. I use to tell my friends my parents were rich. And it was a must that you had groceries. So, when you are raised that way and had to eat what is on your plate, it's hard to tear away from that.

I just kept feeling I needed to change how my family eats and that old way of thinking.

I am officially on to my new lifestyle to go to the grocery store.

Oprah new pictures of her new body pasted everywhere. I bought every copy. I put pictures of that issue in all my cabinets and my 'before' photos on my refrigerator.

My husband said "I am so dang on tired of seeing Oprah everywhere." Get used it. She is here to stay. Of course, I didn't say that out loud.

I think he believed that this was no different from the other million times I tried to lose weight.

I called my doctor's office and asked for a print out of my medical records. I sat there and read every page. If I went in for a cold, they had labeled me as an obese African American. If I had a headache, obese African American. They put that down like it was the reason for all my sickness. I was so bothered by that. I said, "I will never be labeled like that again."

I was really offended by that. I kept thinking about that and I was felt like I was no different than someone on drugs. They are harming there body for the drugs, and I was doing the same thing with food. I said that is it.

I am not really trying to get to a number on the scale. I didn't care about the number on the scale. I wanted to be healthy. I just wanted to get to a place where I felt good on the inside and out. I am not waiting until New Years and not waiting on Monday - that never seems to work to me. No more resolutions and false starts. This time was for keeps.

I was in tears. Oh, it's on. I am gonna do this. I did not tell anyone because this time it was about me. I would wait until everyone was out the house. I would put on my sweats. Although it made me sick to look at myself, but you have to crawl before you walk. So, I had to start in my house. I put on my DVD, and I worked out.

What I could eat - and what I could not - and I followed it just two weeks. I am not kidding. My rings were falling off my fingers. No one noticed, but I was so happy. I knew I had to keep going. Finally, I built up nerves to walk outside.

I begged my daughter and niece to walk with me. They agreed. I could only do it for fifteen minutes. Every week, I would increase my time and add laps. I had already stopped eating bread, rice, potatoes, juice, and sodas. I added whole grain and fiber.

The weight was falling off. People were really complimenting me everywhere we went. I had done so well with walking sometimes I did it twice a day. It was really working.

I joined a gym. I stayed some months, but it was a small one. After carefully logging everything, I noticed that I was losing more weight my way. My kids continued to walk with me, and if they got tired, I told them to sit on the curb and I would still walk.

Within about eight months, I had lost 90 pounds! I was so happy. I would not buy clothes. I just kept sewing up my big clothes. I even had a friend sewing up my clothes. She finally told me to stop bringing her size 24s. She could no longer keep making them into tens and eights. Her advice to me was to go buy some clothes.

I got in my car and cried of joy. I was finally winning this battle. That had me so proud. Finally, I was seeing some results.

I felt like I had not been a good wife. I had not been a good mother. I could never take my kids anywhere. I was always putting it off. Or if we did go, I was not able to buckle my seat belt on the rides. I had made my life miserable and those around me.

It seemed the more weight that I lost, my husband hated it.

I asked, "What's the problem?"

On the phone, it's "I love you, can't wait till you get home from work" and as soon as I walked in the door, you would think that I was the devil. He hated the sight of me.

He told me he thought I was going to lose some weight but not a whole person.

"What is the problem," I asked.

"You look sick to me. You look hungry," he said.

He said that and I started getting upset because he knew I was always sick and tired. Finally, I was feeling better and he was upset! How dare him!

I am finally free of borderline diabetes. I had not had migraines. I am out jumping on the trampoline, playing basketball. I created a better life for me and my kids, and he took a step back from that. He did not want to be a part, so the more he did not like it, the more I wanted to lose.

By this time, my niece was so proud of me, not knowing that she emailed my story in to the Oprah Show. I am at work and they paged me on the intercom. I take the call and was in disbelief that Oprah's producers were on the line. They wanted to hear about my story! Wow! They were going to film me. They called every day. Finally, I asked was it safe to say that I would be on the show. She said yes.

It was crazy. I realized this journey wasn't just for me but to help motivate others. I continued creating ways to shed more weight.

Drinking protein shakes for breakfast sometimes, drinking two if not real hungry and having a big lunch, then adding nuts, almonds, protein bars for snack. I always, always before every meal drink two glasses of water to fill me up and not want seconds or make me thinking of getting something. I helped to eliminate cravings.

I started doing lifting. Five pound and ten pound weights and doing 100 crunches. I did this before I went to bed to keep my metabolism going and burning fat while I was sleep.

I shed 142 pounds in a year and went from a size 24 to a 6.

I felt so good; I was starting to build my confidence up, although it was hard.

Still, I really did not expect for someone to say I look good because I did not know what to say back. It had been ten years since I heard that from anyone. When people would say "OMG, you are so pretty, I would say "So are you."

My friend said "Alicia girl, say thank you."

I worked hard for this, but it is all a process. Can't do it in a day.

Now seeing that my husband and I can not see eye to eye on not one thing, things started to change. I do not know what happened. I tell him I ca not take this. I started seeing my kids act differently because they saw us not getting along.

I told him that I was moving out. The kids and I . Let's see if we can work it out that way. I did not want to give up almost 15 years of marriage. He said let's not do this. The kids need us.

I am determined on moving out, so we decide to sell the house and get an apartment and try. If it didn't work, then we would get a divorce. I sat in my car and I cried because I knew the marriage was over.

I had started building up hate and resentment towards him because I knew that during our marriage, he knew how miserable I was. He knew how sick I was and he knew I did not like the way I looked. I still have the same heart, just a healthier one. Why couldn't he be happy with the new Alicia. The new skinny Alicia.

I thought that I would be healthier, but when you add another 220 pounds of stress, I may as well keep on the 142 pounds I lost. It was less weight, but I was making him happy, not myself.

I had spent almost all of my twenties and some of my thirties miserable in my body. Now, close to 40, I refused to do that for unhealthiness and unhappiness- it's not worth it. I wanted to be happy. If it means we can be happy and be friends apart, then sometimes that is best. I thought about that, then I thought about what everyone around me would say.

When I say I am free of people, because at the end of the day, they are still going to talk about you, whether you are fat, skinny, happy or sad. That is why I am here to tell you when you have been on the emotional roller coaster like I have, you have to start off by loving you again. No one is going to love everything about themselves. There are still things about me I need to work on. I have learned to really love me, not in cocky way, but confident enough to know that I am a child of God and I am who I am for a reason.

I look the way I look for a reason. I remember when I use to hate the way I looked. The Black girls did not like me because they always said I was conceited. I was only being me, but they had to get know me. The White girls that wanted a tanned skin did not like me, so I always had to prove myself. If there was a guy I liked and he was not real cute, he would be insecure. "Why do you like me?" If he was real cute, he was crazy stuff like, "Alicia wants me." It would make people think I was fast. And I wasn't.

All my life, I let things happen. I said as of 2005, I am going to make things happen. There was always a diva in me and it was time to let her out. There is greatness in all of us. How bad do you want it?

Stop staying in a holding pattern. You keep driving in circles. You are close to your destination, but cannot land. Same in your life. What we want is not necessarily what we are supposed to be doing.

There is something. We spend years in negative relationships around so called friends, bringing negative noise. All they come to do is shut you down. They do not believe in themselves. They sure do not believe in you. Trust me, so many people find me, telling me my way of losing weight was wrong, I was walking too slow, all that negative noise.

I am telling you to believe in you so you can land the plane. Quit going in circles. You know you have a vision. That vision was placed in you.

So are you confused or afraid. Once something was placed in you, it was already decided that you are more than able to do it. Remember, we walk by faith not by sight.

Take control of your life. Your situation, only you can do it. The people that are in your life will either grow or go.

When I found myself back in front of the same attorney office, I knew it was time to land the plane as much as it hurt but I knew I wanted him to be happy as well as my self so I had to let the 220 lbs go seemed like all gone in one day. Funny how we hold on to things that really are not meant for us.

What I did to keep it off

I've heard the cliché "failing to plan is planning to fail" at least a million times in my life. I guess I heard it over and over for a reason. The reason is, because it's a true statement. When I decided to make the move toward losing weight, I knew it was going to have to be a lifestyle change versus just a crash diet or temporary fix. I needed to find ways to live this new lifestyle as my truth; I wanted to live in my truth. I've taken some time to jot down the key points that helped me along the way:

- I took control of my life and my situation. That meant being honest with myself and knowing I had been obese before; knowing that the only thing that was going to keep me from going back was me. I know that even if I had a trainer and they could weigh me and tell me all of the healthy things I should eat, I would still leave their office and pig out, especially if I had a stressful day. I had to change my old way of thinking and not make eating my outlet. I had to stop having a pity party for myself, with myself as the only guest. I learned that I am in control of my emotions *and* my eating habits. I began to understand that only I controlled what went in my body. I began to love life, live life and live it in a healthy way.

STRATEGIES THAT WORK FOR ME

• After going through so many obstacles in my life: battling obesity, depression, divorce, strokes, children, border line diabetes, every day life and, God forbid, the dreaded dating life again, I learned that I can overcome any obstacle because I am still here to tell the story. Things are so different now. My best friend told me that she felt like she had to protect me; I was like, "Girl, you must not know dynamite comes in small packages!"

• When I first wake up in the morning I have some quite time to meditate and worship. I learned to say, "I lived my life for everyone else, now I live my life for me and my kids. If I cannot do something, I just say no. Plan your time, instead of doing too much and never completing one task. Learn to journal, that is very important. Never, ever give up on you! Always remember that hot water can boil eggs or soften carrots, which one are you? I used to be the softy that expected to fail and was just going to be a fat, depressed girl forever. But once I stood on my own two feet, I put on my hard shell and I was never giving up on me again. I knew I was ordained to succeed, and so are you.

Stop letting the world tell you, "No." You are what you accept, so what is acceptable to you? Stop letting negative people bring garbage to you, because you are not a trash can. Last, but not least, develop a system. I remember when people saw me walking through my neighborhood and how they had to give me their advice, like I was walking the wrong way at the wrong time, or walk up the hills. Meanwhile, they looked like they should've been out there walking with me. Or perhaps they had lost the weight and gained it back. There was a girl who asked me to help her. She said she wanted to do what I did. I provided her with the system I used. She told me that every 7th day would be her cheat day, but it seemed like every 3rd day was. She would wonder why it wasn't working for her. I advised her that her system was different from mine and she couldn't change it and expect it to work. Just like Wal-mart has a proven system and you don't see any of them closing down, do you? Change what you do in your spare time. Just remember the road to success isn't straight, there are curves called failure, a loop called confusion, speed bumps called friends and red lights called enemies. Caution will have flat times called jobs but have a spare called determination and an engine called perseverance, an insurance called faith and a driver called Jesus there to let you know you will make it and no one will stop you but you. (Author unknown)

Stress-Relieving Strategies That Work For Me

After going through so many obstacles in my life battling obesity, depression, divorce, strokes, children and starting to date again.

I was 21 when I got married. At 37, things are way different.

My best friend Theresa calling me one day and said "Girl I feel like I have to protect you."

I was like, "Girl, dynamite comes in small packages. I am good girl."

- When I get up, I always make some quiet time to worship

- Learn to say no. I think I lived for everyone else. Now, I live for me and my children. If I can't do it, I just say no.

- I was bad at doing so much and not ever finish one thing. Now, I plan my day and my week

- Learn to keep a journal. Very important

- Never give up on you. Remember, hot water can boil eggs or soften carrots. What is in you?

I used to be this softy that accepted I was a failure, which I was going to be fat forever. Once I stood on my own two feet and put my hard shell on, I was not giving up on me ever again. I knew I was ordained to succeed, and so are you. Stop letting the world tell you no. You are what you accept. I decided I would no longer accept being labeled as obese and depressed.

- Start going to motivational speaking events - they are awesome

- Join book clubs. Reading is so important. Open your mind to greatness.

- Stop letting negative people bring garbage to you. You are not a trash can

- I always say develop a system. I remember people use to try and tell me how they lost weight before. I look at them and they had gained the weight back. If your system did not work, I say research. Go to the library, go on the computer. You want to not only learn how to lose weight, but keep it off. That is where system falls in place, like the larger restaurant.

- Like McDonald's, all the places now going out of business, how many McDonald have you seen go out of business? There is a system they follow, and there are no cutting corners. This one lady told me I will do your plan but every 7th day is my cheat day so seem like every three days I talked to her she was on her cheat day I just told her that's your system not mind you can't change the system that works.

1.) You can't change the people you take advice from.

2.) Change what you do in your spare time.

- Just remember this: The road to success is not straight. There are curves called failure, a loop called confusion, speed bumps called friends, red lights called enemies, caution will have flats, called job but I have a spare called determination, an engine called perseverance, insurance called faith and a driver called Jesus. I will make it and no one will stop me but me! (Author unknown)

- Set times you eat and try to stick with it these are times.

    - 2 glasses water soon as you wake up

    - 7:00 protein shakes

    - 10:30 protein 2 glass or water

    - 1:30 salad or grilled chicken vegetables maybe fruit

    - 4:30 fruit almonds yogurt two glasses of water

    - 7:30 grilled or baked meat vegetables

3.) Upon walking make time to meditate

4.) Know that this is a lifestyle you want to master.

5.) God is the master

6.) I can master all things through him

7.) Know your body

8.) Talk to your doctor

9.) Ask questions

10.) Ask for copies of your medical records.

11.) Learn what different food groups are

12.) Change your eating habits

13.) Replace them with the right choices

14.) Don't make it difficult, its not. I don't even entertain the thought waiter bring bread to the table no thank you.

15.) Get your rest

- Learn to keep your body and mind rejuvenated

- Take bubble baths

- When I first get home from work, I take 30 minute breather

16.) Exercise

17.) Journal

- Keep up with what you do daily so you can track your progress

Monday
Breakfast
Snack
Lunch
Snack
Dinner
Snack
Water intake
Exercise
What do you think you should have done different?
Did you do your best this week

Track Your Success

This Weeks Weight_____   Goal Weight _____

Breakfast   _____

Snack   _____

Lunch   _____

Snack   _____

Dinner   _____

Water intake   _____

Daily Exercise   _____

How are you doing?   _____

_____

_____

What changes have you made to help your
transformation?   _____

_____

_____

_____

_____

Track Your Success

This Weeks Weight_____   Goal Weight _____

Breakfast   _____

Snack   _____

Lunch   _____

Snack   _____

Dinner   _____

Water intake   _____

Daily Exercise   _____

How are you doing?   _____

_____

_____

What changes have you made to help your
transformation?   _____

_____

_____

_____

_____

Track Your Success

This Weeks Weight_____   Goal Weight _____

Breakfast   _____

Snack   _____

Lunch   _____

Snack   _____

Dinner   _____

Water intake   _____

Daily Exercise   _____

How are you doing?   _____

_____

_____

What changes have you made to help your
transformation?   _____

_____

_____

_____

_____

Track Your Success

This Weeks Weight_____   Goal Weight _____

Breakfast   _____

Snack   _____

Lunch   _____

Snack   _____

Dinner   _____

Water intake   _____

Daily Exercise   _____

How are you doing?   _____

_____

_____

What changes have you made to help your
transformation?   _____

_____

_____

_____

_____

Track Your Success

This Weeks Weight_____   Goal Weight _____

Breakfast   _____

Snack   _____

Lunch   _____

Snack   _____

Dinner   _____

Water intake   _____

Daily Exercise   _____

How are you doing?   _____

_____

_____

What changes have you made to help your
transformation?   _____

_____

_____

_____

_____

Track Your Success

This Weeks Weight_____   Goal Weight _____

Breakfast   _____

Snack   _____

Lunch   _____

Snack   _____

Dinner   _____

Water intake   _____

Daily Exercise   _____

How are you doing?   _____

_____

_____

What changes have you made to help your
transformation?   _____

_____

_____

_____

_____

Track Your Success

This Weeks Weight_____   Goal Weight _____

Breakfast   _____

Snack   _____

Lunch   _____

Snack   _____

Dinner   _____

Water intake   _____

Daily Exercise   _____

How are you doing?   _____

_____

_____

What changes have you made to help your
transformation?   _____

_____

_____

_____

_____

Track Your Success

This Weeks Weight_____   Goal Weight _____

Breakfast   _____

Snack   _____

Lunch   _____

Snack   _____

Dinner   _____

Water intake   _____

Daily Exercise   _____

How are you doing?   _____

_____

_____

What changes have you made to help your
transformation?   _____

_____

_____

_____

_____

Suggested Meals

MONDAY

BREAKFAST
1 scrambled egg
1 tablespoon low fat cheese
1 orange cut in slices

LUNCH
1 can tuna
chopped celery
1 tablespoon sesame oil
1/8 teaspoon dill and lemon pepper
sliced tomato

SNACK
1 cup of berries or orange slices
½ cup mixed nuts

DINNER
broiled salmon
olive oil
½ cup brown rice
½ cup steamed broccoli

SNACK
¾ cup plain yogurt

TUESDAY

BREAKFAST
chocolate protein shake
soy milk or water
crushed ice in blender
1 banana
1 tablespoon of orange Metamucil (fiber)

SNACK
1/2 grapefruit

LUNCH
2 cups lettuce
¼ tomatoes
bell pepper
low fat cheese
1 diced hardboiled egg
2 tablespoons lemon juice
2 teaspoons olive oil
½ slice whole grain toast or pita bread

DINNER
nude burger (no bread)
boca burger
2 slices tomatoes
1 slice onion
½ cup string beans
½ medium orange

SNACK
10 almonds

WEDNESDAY

BREAKFAST
1 cup oatmeal (fruit on top if you like)
1 cup fat free milk

SNACK
protein bar

LUNCH
2 ounces roast chicken breast
¼ cup each lettuce tomatoes
1 slice wheat bread
½ cup berries

SNACK
apple topped with peanut butter

DINNER
5 ounces baked chicken breast
2 cups mixed zucchini and squash sauteed in 1 teaspoon
olive oil with seasoning of your likings

SNACK
½ cup berries

THURSDAY

BREAKFAST
4 ounces lean turkey sausage sauteed with sliced onion and pepper in 1 teaspoon of olive oil
1 sliced tomato

SNACK
1 nectarine

LUNCH
grilled chicken salad
1 egg
1 tomato
½ pineapple
low fat cheese

SNACK
protein bar

DINNER
2 baked fish topped with lemon
steamed broccoli
½ cup medium oranges

SNACK
1 cup of yogurt

FRIDAY

BREAKFAST
strawberry protein shake
water or soy milk crushed ice
1 banana
½ cup strawberries
1 tablespoon orange Metamucil (fiber)

SNACK
1/2 cup almonds

LUNCH
1 slice toasted whole wheat bread topped with tuna
1 cup fruit
15 steamed baby carrots

SNACK
1 cup yogurt

DINNER
2 baked pork chops
1cup sauteed veggies in 1 teaspoon olive oil
1 cup steamed brown rice

SNACK
1 pear

SATURDAY

BREAKFAST

2 slices turkey bacon

1 scrambled egg

1 slice whole grain toast

SNACK

1 apple sliced topped with peanut butter

LUNCH

5 ounces chicken breast

2 cups mixed zucchini and squash sauteed with olive oil, lightly seasoned

SNACK

protein bar

DINNER

lemon pepper chicken

½ cup steamed broccoli

½ cup baby carrots

2 Wasa crackers

SNACK

1 cup seedless grapes

SUNDAY

BREAKFAST
bowl oatmeal
orange slices

SNACK
½ cup oranges
1 cup yogurt

LUNCH
2 baked fish topped with lemon slices
steamed veggies of your choice

SNACK
1 cup oranges

DINNER
lemon pepper chicken
½ cup brown rice
steamed broccoli

SNACK
1 pear

MONDAY

BREAKFAST
protein shake

SNACK
1 pear
1ounce mozzarella cheese

LUNCH
salad
lettuce with tuna
sliced tomatoes
bell pepper
2 Wasa crackers
mixed fruit

SNACK
½ cup mixed nuts

DINNER
2 ounces turkey
¼ cup low fat feta cheese
2 cups lettuce
½ cup tomatoes
½ cucumber
5 olives
2 tbs fat free vinaigrette
1 whole wheat pita
10 grapes

SNACK
100 calorie snack thin crisps

TUESDAY

BREAKFAST
2 turkey bacon slices
1 wheat toast
1 egg poached

SNACK
sliced grapefruit

LUNCH
2 ounces baked chicken breast
1 tablespoon orange marmalade
1 teaspoon Dijon mustard
2/3 cup couscous tossed with ½ cup broccoli

SNACK
1 cup yogurt

DINNER
protein shake

SNACK
pear

WEDNESDAY

BREAKFAST
1 cup yogurt
1 tablespoon low fat granola
1 cup mixed fruit

SNACK
protein bar

LUNCH
protein shake

SNAKE
apple slices with peanut butter

DINNER
5 ounces baked chicken breast
½ cup string beans
½ cup brown rice
½ orange

SNACK
½ cup berries

FITNESS TIPS

- Make sure you get enough Omega 3 fatty acids. I take them in the form of flax seed oil. Research shows that Omega 3 fatty acids are great for controlling hunger, regulating blood sugar, stress and hormone levels - all of which contributes to excess flab.

- Take a good multi-vitamin. I also take 1200 milligrams of Calcium. This mineral helps to increase fat burning by up to 70%. It also strengthens your bones.

- I love herbal teas. When have late night energy to snack get a cup of tea there are so many flavors to choose from. I keep about 5 different flavors on hand. I add ½ teaspoon of Splenda Herbal teas can help to relax you, plus they are filling and soothing.

- Drink two (2) eight ounce glasses of water before every meal, and two to three more throughout the day. This works great for your skin and helps give you a full feeling to stop the cravings and overeating.

- Exercise is a must. I live by the crawl, walk, run method. Start slow if you are not that active. Do what your body will allow. Keep in mind that the more you do, the better the results. If you have been inactive for a while, start off with 15 minutes of walking. Good ways to do this include: start parking further away when running errands, taking the stairs instead of elevators or escalators.

- When at home, get up and walk in place during the commercial breaks.

- Consider investing in a 5 pound weight to use during your favorite show.

- After a couple of weeks, you should be able to walk for 25 to 30 minutes.

- Thirty to 45 days into your new lifestyle, you should be able to jog. Don't cheat yourself - you must be held accountable to your healthy lifestyle.

- Gradually increase the duration of your workouts from 30 minutes to 45 minutes, then to one hour. Pick up the pace with your running and use weights for 20 minutes, 3 to 4 times a week.

- Every night before I go to bed, I do two minutes of leg lunges up and down the hall, 100 crunches and 10 minutes of light weights to keep the metabolism going and burn fat as I sleep.

God First is the Key to Reaching Your Goals!

My faith in God is what kept me. Every day that I put my two feet on the pavement to walk, I would repeat Philippians 4:13, "I can do all things through Christ who strengthens me." I said that verse so much, I was walking and preaching to myself and I had it broken down. Now in the Word it says *all*, so I was not going to limit myself anymore to what I could do. The Word also says *I can do*, so I had to realize only *I* can do this. Nobody could walk for me or eat for me, only I could. It said *through Christ*, which meant I had to have a relationship with Him to get to that point of reaching my goals and not going back to that unhealthy lifestyle. Even when I would get to a place that was really troubling, I created that atmosphere of walking and it was good for my body *and* my soul.

Like most people, my grandmother was a very spiritual matriarch for my family. I can remember being brought up in the church. My grandmother, Mrs. Cluster Turner, and her neighbor, Gladys Mathis, are Christians for real. I used to think they had God's phone number—they knew everything.

When I say they have been best friends forever, I mean I have never seen them get upset with each other or let a curse word slip out of their mouths. I couldn't believe this was true.

I am a Christian, but every now and then, you mess with a woman, especially a Black woman's kids, and you are getting ready to be told off. We cannot handle that. But my grandmother was my rock and my shield. I could go to her whenever I needed to vent or get some spiritual advice about something that was bothering me or wearing on my spiritual inner man.

She wouldn't mind getting her good girlfriends on a prayer circle either. She knew the importance of having that connection with God and being able to freely communicate with Him. Allowing His holy spirit to flow in the medium and reveal things to you. Through this insight we are in turn able to deal with otherwise unimaginable situations. God is there for us to call upon in our good and bad times. So this I say to you: Keep God on speed dial.

DEAR OPRAH

After receiving my O magazine for the month, I was in tears. I was in tears for so many reasons. One of the major reasons I was in tears was because I, too, had struggled with being overweight. I was embarrassed and depressed for so many years. I had felt the disgrace of losing a few pounds only to gain it back again. I felt shame for going back and forth and being on a diet roller coaster. It just became embarrassing to mention to anyone that I was dieting. I felt like if I didn't tell anyone that I wouldn't let anyone down, including myself. After seeing you finally lose the weight and seeing the smile on your face the day you walked out showing the world you had won! Most people would die to win the GRAMMY or an OSCAR, but you had won the battle of obesity. It's a battle that so many people feel like they will never ever achieve because it is hard to overcome. It is comparable to being a drug addict, and you did it in front of millions of people.

Oprah, you are the one who motivated me to lose 142 pounds. This is something that I have tried to do over the last 10 years. I tried over and over again, and until I saw that you did it, that is when things started to turn around for me. I plastered all of your skinny photos in my cupboards. Funny how people put stuff up on the bathroom mirror, but in this case, I needed to put it where I knew I would see it—where the food was! Every time I thought about cheating, you were there looking at me as if you were saying, "Girl, don't do it." I thought about how successful you are and all that you have overcome to get where you are now. I have had some pretty hard blows in life—a divorce after a fifteen-year marriage, losing my job, my home, and basically living out of my car. Food became my husband, my home, my job, and my comfort. But I am here to tell you, Oprah, I am an emotional eate,r and I did not know that until after being on your show and Bob Greene kept asking me why was I overweight before. He said that for most people it's a reason—abusive marriage or something. I was looking at him like look there is no other reason except that I like to eat, and then after going through the divorce that's when it hit me that I was an emotional eater. My then husband didn't like the weight loss, and I almost slipped back to that emotional depressed person that I used to be because I was a people pleaser. It was from that moment on that I realized that I would please myself and turn my negative habits into positive ones. I went from eating ice cream to yogurt. Instead of eating chocolate, I would grab a protein bar. If I wanted a milk shake, I would make a protein shake. If I was unhappy and felt that I didn't please someone, I would dress up and tell my daughter to get the camera and come on have a photo shoot with me. We would have so much fun just taking pictures of ourselves and reaffirming that we were beautiful on the inside and the OUTSIDE. Some people would say that I love the camera, but I am confident enough to say that I love me! I was tired of having a pity party all those years. I was fat, miserabl,e and mad because everyone else was skinny and happy. At least, that's how I saw everyone else. Enough was enough. I said that I would never again have a pity party. I became the love of my life and transformed from the inside out. I decided that I loved myself enough not to go back.

Oprah, you were and still are my motivation to losing the weight and becoming a voice to so many others that struggle with the same mental and physical strongholds of weight loss. I love you Oprah for who you are and what you have done for so many others and me. You are beautiful inside and out. Don't be embarrassed or hard on yourself because,e like you said, you know what to do and realizing that its about you and how you feel and what makes Oprah happy—whether it's a size 4 OR a size 14. TRULY, THE NUMBER ON THE SCALE DOES NOT MATTER. IT'S WHAT YOU FEEL ON THE INSIDE AND THAT WILL FLOW OUT.

With sincere love,

Alicia Ash

About the Author

Alicia Ash is a Motivational Speaker and Author of the new self-improvement book, "I Dropped 142 lbs in a Year and Lost 220 lbs in a Day." Born Alicia Lannette in Dothan,Alabama, Ash has been a featured guest on numerous television and radio shows, most notably the "Oprah Winfrey Show", and has penned expositions in the Atlanta Journal Constitution newspaper, Columbus Times newspaper and Women World Magazine on the affects of weight gain and loss and, its impact on self, family, faith and finances. Prior to her journey of healthy living, Alicia suffered three strokes in a years' time frame, as well as bouts of depression . It was after one of her strokes when doctors informed her that she was borderline Diabetic and that a drastic change in her eating habits and lifestyle were imperative to her continuing to live. It was after hearing that dreadful report that Alicia was motivated by the fear of not being able to see her children grow up that she changed her life forever. She would go on to change her diet to a strict regiment as well as add exercising daily to her daily lifestyle.

These days one can find Alicia busy on the lecture circuit speaking at conferences for women's groups and at health and fitness workshops about her life story. The collective maltreatment encourages Ash to be unwavering in her mission to empower, inform and boost the confidence of all those she encounters, while on the road. She has encountered a great amount of support and appreciation from fans around the country, consistently telling her how she has helped them to changed their lives or how she has motivated them to start taking their health and diet seriously. The devoted and proud mother of two, daughter Merceytee (17) and son William (10), claims them as her main motivating factor to changing her life. On top of that, she says that she feels God has blessed her to be in this position for a reason. With that in mind, Alicia is starting a foundation called "Skin Deep Foundation", which will be devoted to using the skin left over from surgical procedures to being donated to burn victims whom are in need for their surgeries. She said the idea came to her after she lost the 142lbs and was dealing with having all of that skin removed herself. She is currently looking into the research involved with the medical practicality of collecting skin removed from surgery and the ability to be able to reuse that skin.

The book chronicles Alicia's experiences during the time period of being her heaviest to losing the weight, both the good and bad. Like the fact that her husband of 15 years was no longer attracted to her after she lost all of the weight, because he felt strongly about not being physically attracted to her because she was a small frame woman. She says that was probably the hardest thing to deal with emotionally, because she never envisioned losing her husband as a part of the pitfalls of losing the weight. The book will be in stores and available online shortly, and she plans to embark on a book tour to support the book once it hits stores.

For booking appearances, book signings, interviews and/or sponsorship opportunities contact Carlos Scott/ N-Vision Marketing Inc at 404-484-7306 or nvisioninc1@ gmail.com.

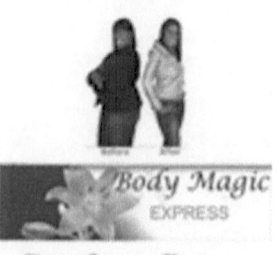

Body Magic
EXPRESS

CALL JERRY BUTLER

(757) 971 - 3733

www.ardysslife.com/jerrybutler

<u>LET JERRY BUTLER REPAIR YOUR CREDIT NOW!!!
AS LOW AS $25.00 DOWN!!!
WOULD YOU LIKE TO IMPROVE YOUR CREDIT RATING BY
REMOVING THOSE NEGATIVES FROM
"YOUR" CREDIT REPORT?
LOWER YOUR HOUSE PAYMENTS UP TO $500.00 A MONTH
WITH A LOAN MODIFICATION!!!
ASK ME HOW TO GET "YOUR" CREDIT REPAIRED "FREE"!!!
HOW TO GET "YOUR" WEBSITE AND PAGE CUSTOMIZED "FREE"!!!
HOW TO DRIVE "MORE" TRAFFIC TO "YOUR" SITE "FREE"!!!
HOW TO GET "YOUR" BODYMAGIC OUTFIT ABSOLUTELY "FREE"!!!</u>

BUSINESS OWNERS, ENTREPRENEURS, SIGNED & UNSIGNED ARTIST CAN NOW ADVERTISE THEIR BUSINESS OVER THE AIRWAVES TO MILLIONS ABSOLUTELY "FREE"!!!... SIMPLY GO TO BLACKSTARTUPBIZ.COM... SIGN UP TO BE A GUEST...THEN CALL JERRY BUTLER AT 757 971 FREE (3733)...OR EMAIL ME AT ASKJERRYB2004@AOL.COM

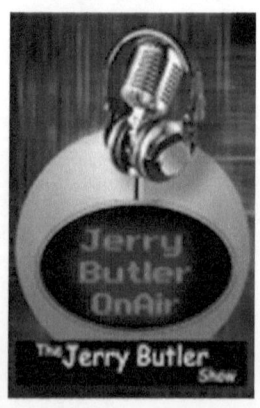

OUR GOAL is to INSPIRE people of EVERY Race,Creed and Color to be THE VERY BEST THEY CAN BE!!!

www.ingramcontent.com/pod-product-compliance
Lightning Source LLC
Chambersburg PA
CBHW020245290526
45784CB00003B/1102